Management of Neck Pain

Guest Editor

ALLEN SINCLAIR CHEN, MD, MPH

PHYSICAL MEDICINE AND REHABILITATION CLINICS OF NORTH AMERICA

www.pmr.theclinics.com

Consulting Editor
GEORGE H. KRAFT, MD, MS

August 2011 • Volume 22 • Number 3

SAUNDERS an imprint of ELSEVIER, Inc.

W.B. SAUNDERS COMPANY
A Division of Elsevier Inc.

1600 John F. Kennedy Boulevard ● Suite 1800 ● Philadelphia, Pennsylvania 19103

http://www.theclinics.com

PHYSICAL MEDICINE AND REHABILITATION CLINICS OF NORTH AMERICA Volume 22, Number 3 August 2011 ISSN 1047-9651, ISBN-13: 978-1-4557-1121-5

Editor: Debora Dellapena
Developmental Editor: Donald Mumford

Reprints. For copies of 100 or more of articles in this publication, please contact the Commercial Reprints Department, Elsevier Inc., 360 Park Avenue South, New York, NY 10010-1710. Tel.: 212-633-3812; Fax: 212-462-1935; E-mail: reprints@elsevier.com.

Physical Medicine and Rehabilitation Clinics of North America (ISSN 1047-9651) is published quarterly by Elsevier Inc., 360 Park Avenue South, New York, NY 10010-1710. Months of issue are February, May, August, and November. Business and Editorial Offices: 1600 John F. Kennedy Blvd., Suite 1800, Philadelphia, PA 19103-2899. Customer Service Office: 3251 Riverport Lane, Maryland Heights, MO 63043. Periodicals postage paid at New York, NY and additional mailing offices. Subscription price per year is $230.00 (US individuals), $414.00 (US institutions), $122.00 (US students), $280.00 (Canadian individuals), $540.00 (Canadian institutions), $175.00 (Canadian students), $345.00 (foreign individuals), $540.00 (foreign institutions), and $175.00 (foreign students). Foreign air speed delivery is included in all *Clinics* subscription prices. All prices are subject to change without notice. **POSTMASTER:** Send address changes to *Physical Medicine and Rehabilitation Clinics of North America*, Customer Service Office: Elsevier Health Sciences Division, Subscription Customer Service, 3251 Riverport Lane, Maryland Heights, MO 63043. **Customer Service: 1-800-654-2452 (US). From outside of the United States, call 314-447-8871. Fax: 314-447-8029. E-mail: JournalsCustomer Service-usa@elsevier.com (for print support); JournalsOnlineSupport-usa@elsevier.com (for online support).**

Physical Medicine and Rehabilitation Clinics of North America is indexed in *Excerpta Medica, MEDLINE/ PubMed (Index Medicus), Cinahl,* and *Cumulative Index to Nursing and Allied Health Literature.*

Printed and bound by CPI Group (UK) Ltd, Croydon, CR0 4YY

Transferred to Digital Print 2011

Contributors

CONSULTING EDITOR

GEORGE H. KRAFT, MD, MS
Alvord Professor of Multiple Sclerosis Research; Professor, Department of Rehabilitation Medicine, and Adjunct Professor, Department of Neurology, University of Washington, Seattle, Washington

GUEST EDITOR

ALLEN SINCLAIR CHEN, MD, MPH
Interventional Spine, Department of Physical Medicine and Rehabilitation, The Permanente Medical Group, Martinez, California

AUTHORS

ERIC P. ALEXANDER, MD
Department of Physical Medicine and Rehabilitation; Associate Chief, The Permanente Medical Group, Martinez, California

DANIEL ALVES, MD
Physiatrist, Universal Pain Management, Los Angeles, California

RAHUL BASHO, MD
Attending Spinal Surgeon, Riverside County Regional Medical Center, Riverside, California

AMANDEEP BHALLA, MD
Resident, Department of Orthopaedic Surgery, Harbor–University of California, Los Angeles, Los Angeles, California

NIKOLAI BOGDUK, MD, PhD, DSc, MMed, FAFRM, FFPM (ANZCA)
Conjoint Professor of Pain Medicine, Newcastle Bone and Joint Institute, Royal Newcastle Centre, University of Newcastle, New South Wales, Australia

MARIA CARPINTERO, MD
Fellow, Division of Rheumatology, Department of Internal Medicine, University of Miami Miller School of Medicine, Miami, Florida

MARY SUSAN CHEN, PT, GCFP
Midwest Representative of the Feldenkrais Guild, Private Practice, River Forest, Chicago, Illinois

LEAH G. CONCANNON, MD
Fellow, Department of Rehabilitation Medicine, University of Washington, Seattle, Washington

DEBORAH DARR, PT
Deborah Darr Physical Therapy; Rehabilitation Institute of Chicago Center for Pain Management, Chicago, Illinois

DAVID E. FISH, MD, MPH
Chief, Division of Interventional Physiatry; Assistant Professor, Department of Orthopaedics, Physical Medicine and Rehabilitation, The UCLA Spine Center, David Geffen School of Medicine at University of California, Los Angeles, Santa Monica, California

ALFRED C. GELLHORN, MD
Clinical Assistant Professor, Departments of Rehabilitation Medicine and Orthopedics and Sports Medicine, University of Washington, Seattle, Washington

BRETT A. GERSTMAN, MD
UCLA/WLA VA PM&R Pain Medicine Fellowship Program, David Geffen School of Medicine at University of California, Los Angeles; Department of Physical Medicine and Rehabilitation, Los Angeles, California

AVIVA HOPKINS, MD
Fellow, Division of Rheumatology, Department of Internal Medicine, University of Miami Miller School of Medicine, Miami, Florida

ANAND B. JOSHI, MD, MHA
Penn Spine Center, University of Pennsylvania, Philadelphia, Pennsylvania

SAMANTHA L. KANAREK, DO, MS
Resident, Rehabilitation Medicine, University of Washington, Seattle, Washington

VISHAL KANCHERLA, DO
Physiatrist, Austin Diagnostic Clinic, Austin, Texas

NATASHA KIM, DC
Carmel, Indiana

BRIAN J. KRABAK, MD, MBA
Clinical Associate Professor, Rehabilitation, Orthopaedics and Sports Medicine, University of Washington and Seattle Children's Sports Medicine; Physician, University of Washington and Seattle University Athletics; Team Physician, USA Swimming; Medical Director, Racing The Planet Ultra-Marathons, Seattle, Washington

SCOTT R. LAKER, MD
Clinical Assistant Professor, Departments of Rehabilitation Medicine and Orthopedics and Sports Medicine, University of Washington, Seattle, Washington

REBECCA LANSKY, DO
Department of Physical Medicine and Rehabilitation, University of Pennsylvania, Philadelphia, Pennsylvania

PAUL C. LEE, MD
Resident Physician, University of California, Los Angeles/Veterans Affairs Greater Los Angeles Multicampus Physical Medicine and Rehabilitation Residency Program; Department of Physical Medicine and Rehabilitation Greater Los Angeles Veterans Affairs, Los Angeles, California

VICTORIA LIN, MSIV
David Geffen School of Medicine at University of California Los Angeles; Office of the Dean-Student Affairs, Los Angeles, California

AI MUKAI, MD
Physiatrist, Texas Orthopedics Sports and Rehabilitation, Austin, Texas

ELANA M. OBERSTEIN, MD, MPH, FACR
Arthritis and Rheumatic Disease Specialties, Aventura, Florida

GLENN OZOA, DO
Physiatrist, Beverly Hills Orthopedic Group, Beverly Hills, California

SANJOG PANGARKAR, MD
Director, Inpatient Pain Service, Veterans Health Service Greater Los Angeles; Assistant Clinical Professor, David Geffen School of Medicine at University of California, Los Angeles; Department of Physical Medicine and Rehabilitation Greater Los Angeles Veterans Affairs, Los Angeles, California

CHRISTOPHER T. PLASTARAS, MD
Department of Physical Medicine and Rehabilitation, Penn Spine Center, University of Pennsylvania, Philadelphia, Pennsylvania

SETH SCHRAN, MD
Department of Physical Medicine and Rehabilitation, Penn Spine Center, University of Pennsylvania, Philadelphia, Pennsylvania

SUSAN SOROSKY, MD
Desert Spine and Sports Physicians, Phoenix, Arizona

JEFFREY WANG, MD
Professor of Orthopaedic Surgery and Neurosurgery, UCLA Spine Center, University of California, Los Angeles School of Medicine, Santa Monica, California

STEVE H. YOON, MD
Kerlan-Jobe Orthopaedic Clinic, Los Angeles, California

Contents

Neck pain should not, and must not, be confused with cervical radicular pain. Equating the two conditions, or confusing them, results in misdiagnosis, inappropriate investigations, and inappropriate treatment that is destined to fail. So critical is the difference that pedagogically it is unwise to include the two topics in the same book, let alone the same article. However, traditions and expectations are hard to break. In deference to habit, this article addresses both entities, but does so by underplaying cervical radicular pain so as to retain the emphasis on neck pain.

Neck pain is a common and costly problem in Western society. Nearly two-thirds of the US population will experience neck pain at some point in their lives, and at any one time about 5% of the US population has sufficient neck pain to cause disability. Although the likelihood of defining a precise cause of neck pain is low, if the etiology and structural source can be determined, they may be valuable in directing treatment. Patient history serves to identify red flags and yellow flags, whereas the physical examination, guided by the history, serves primarily to confirm those suspicions.

Neck and shoulder pain are common complaints among the general population, being the second and third most common musculoskeletal complaints, respectively, after back pain in the primary care setting. Differentiating between neck and shoulder pain can be challenging, as both share symptoms and physical examination findings. The differential diagnoses of neck and shoulder pain are extensive. Providers are encouraged to develop a systematic, comprehensive, and reproducible approach, including thorough history taking and physical examination along with focused diagnostic testing.

The patient with neck pain may pose a diagnostic dilemma for the treating physician. As with other areas of medicine, imaging is guided by the history and physical examination. The steady advance of 3-dimensional, functional, and nuclear medicine studies make it increasingly important that the ordering physician be aware of the potential benefits and disadvantages of imaging options. This article reviews the current literature on imaging for the patient with neck pain, illustrates several imaging abnormalities, and discusses the workup of commonly seen patient populations.

involves injury to the neurovascular structures in the cervicobrachial region. A classification system based on etiology, symptoms, clinical presentation, and anatomy is supported by most physicians. The first type of TOS is vascular, involving compression of either the subclavian artery or vein. The second type is true neurogenic TOS, which involves injury to the brachial plexus. Finally, the third and most controversial type is referred to as disputed neurogenic TOS. This article aims to provide the reader some understanding of the pathophysiology, workup, and treatment of this fascinating clinical entity.

This article provides a comprehensive review of rheumatologic considerations for a clinician when evaluating a patient with neck pain. Clearly, anatomic derangements of the cervical spine should be considered when a patient complains of cervicalgia. However, one must also entertain the possibility of a systemic illness as the cause of the pain. Examples of diseases that may present with a prominent feature of neck pain are discussed, including rheumatoid arthritis, ankylosing spondylitis, diffuse idiopathic skeletal hyperostosis, myositis, and fibromyalgia. Evidence of an underlying rheumatic illness may guide the clinician in a different therapeutic direction.

This article offers conservative treatment strategies for patients suffering from musculoskeletal causes of neck pain. Basic pharmacology is reviewed, including that of opioids, nonsteroidal anti-inflammatory drugs, adjuvants, and topical analgesics. Moreover, indications for therapeutic exercise, manual therapy, and modalities are reviewed, along with any supporting literature. Treatment considerations with each category of medication and physical therapy are discussed. This article is meant to serve as a resource for physicians to tailor conservative treatment options to their individual patients.

Of the multitude of treatment options for the management of neck pain, no obvious single treatment modality has been shown to be most efficacious. As such, the clinician should consider alternative treatment modalities if a modality is engaging, available, financially feasible, potentially efficacious, and is low risk for the patient. As evidence-based medicine for neck pain develops, the clinician is faced with the challenge of which treatments to encourage patients to pursue. Treatment modalities explored in this article, including chiropractic, acupuncture, TENS, massage, yoga, Tai Chi, and Feldenkrais, represent reasonable complementary and alternative medicine methods for patients with neck pain.

Percutaneous interventional spinal procedures have become ubiquitous in the management of cervical pain syndromes. This article reviews the indications, contraindications, patient selection, and potential complications of epidural injections, zygapophyseal joint and medial branch nerve injections, spinal cord stimulation, and radiofrequency neurotomy.

Through the myriad of abnormalities encountered by spine surgeons, neck pain is one of the most perplexing. The nature, onset, and location of the pain all provide information as to what the potential pain generator may be. By synthesizing data garnered from the physical examination, imaging studies, and history, a spine surgeon must formulate a differential diagnosis and treatment plan. The surgeon must determine whether the patient has cervical radiculopathy, myelopathy, or simply cervical spondylosis because the treatment of each of these is vastly different.

THE CLINICS ARE NOW AVAILABLE ONLINE!

Access your subscription at:
www.theclinics.com

Preface

Management of Neck Pain

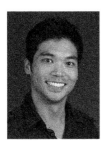

Allen Sinclair Chen, MD, MPH
Guest Editor

With variable pain generators and differing responses to treatment, neck pain can pose a challenging problem for both patients and providers. Diagnostic evaluations, which include electrodiagnosis and radiologic imaging, can help evaluate underlying pathophysiology, but often do not correlate with symptomatology.

Among the myriad of treatment options, many lack strong supporting evidence, rendering the management of neck and associated radicular pain even more difficult. As such, the art of medicine and the physician-patient relationship become particularly crucial in determining proper, safe, and effective evaluation and treatment for this common complaint.

I am honored that Dr George Kraft, a teacher and mentor to me for several years, invited me to guest edit this *Physical Medicine and Rehabilitation Clinics of North America* issue devoted to neck pain. My aim was to present a clear and organized approach to the topic, and I am very fortunate to have gathered a truly outstanding and talented panel of contributors from around the world, and from diverse medical backgrounds.

Together, these accomplished authors have provided the reader with a concise and accurate understanding of anatomy, evaluation, and treatment options for neck and associated radicular pain. I am pleased with their individual contributions and with this issue as a whole.

Allen Sinclair Chen, MD, MPH
Interventional Spine
Department of Physical Medicine and Rehabilitation
The Permanente Medical Group
Diablo Service Area
200 Muir Road, Hacienda Building
Martinez, CA 94553, USA

Phys Med Rehabil Clin N Am 22 (2011) xiii
doi:10.1016/j.pmr.2011.04.002   pmr.theclinics.com
1047-9651/11/$ – see front matter © 2011 Elsevier Inc. All rights reserved.

The Anatomy and Pathophysiology of Neck Pain

Nikolai Bogduk, MD, PhD, DSc, MMed, FAFRM, FFPM (ANZCA)

KEYWORDS

• Neck pain • Cervical • Anatomy • Nerve supply

In preparation for considering the pathophysiology of neck pain, a critical distinction must be made. The neck is not the upper limb. The upper limb is not the neck. By the same token, pain in the neck is not pain in the upper limb, and vice versa.

For these reasons, neck pain should not, and must not, be confused with cervical radicular pain. Neck pain is perceived in the neck, and its causes, mechanisms, investigation, and treatment are different from those of cervical radicular pain. Reciprocally, cervical radicular pain is perceived in the upper limb, and its causes, mechanisms, investigation, and treatment are different from those of neck pain. Equating the 2 conditions, or confusing them, results in misdiagnosis, inappropriate investigations, and inappropriate treatment that is destined to fail.

Confusion arises because neck pain and cervical radicular pain are both caused by disorders of the cervical spine, but this common site of disease does not constitute a basis for equating the 2 conditions. In all other respects the 2 conditions are totally different.

So critical is the difference that pedagogically it is unwise to include the 2 topics in the same book, let alone the same article. Doing so, as has been the tradition, risks readers remaining confused, and applying to neck pain the interpretations, investigations, and treatment that apply to radicular pain. However, traditions and expectations are difficult to break. In deference to habit, this article addresses both entities, but does so by underplaying cervical radicular pain so as to retain the emphasis on neck pain. Cervical radicular pain is covered in a later article, and more comprehensively elsewhere.[1]

RADICULAR PAIN

Perhaps surprisingly, but nonetheless veritably, little is known about the causes and mechanisms of cervical radicular pain. In the literature, cervical radicular pain has

The author has nothing to disclose.
Newcastle Bone and Joint Institute, Royal Newcastle Centre, University of Newcastle, PO Box 664J, Newcastle, New South Wales 2300, Australia
E-mail address: vicki.caesar@hnehealth.nsw.gov.au

conventionally been addressed in the context of cervical radiculopathy; but radiculopathy is not synonymous with radicular pain.

Cervical radiculopathy is a neurologic condition characterized by objective signs of loss of neurologic function: some combination of sensory loss, motor loss, or impaired reflexes, in a segmental distribution. None of these features constitutes pain.

Many causes of cervical radiculopathy have been reported (**Table 1**). They share the common feature that they compress or otherwise compromise a cervical spinal nerve or its roots. The axons of these nerves are either compressed directly or are rendered ischemic by compression of their blood supply. Symptoms of sensory or motor loss arise as a result of block of conduction along the affected axons. The features of cervical radiculopathy, therefore, are essentially negative in nature; they reflect loss of function. In contrast, pain is a positive feature, not caused by loss of nerve function.

For this reason cervical radicular pain cannot be summarily attributed to the same causes as those of radiculopathy. Compression of axons does not elicit pain. If compression is to be invoked as a mechanism for pain it must explicitly relate to compression of a dorsal root ganglion.

Laboratory experiments on lumbar nerve roots have shown that mechanical compression of nerve roots does not elicit activity in nociceptive afferent fibers.[2,3] Therefore, compression of nerve roots cannot be held to be the mechanism of radicular pain. However, compression of a dorsal root ganglion does evoke sustained

Table 1
Possible causes of cervical radiculopathy, listed by structure and condition

Structure	Condition
Intervertebral disc	Protrusion
	Herniation
	Osteophytes
Zygapophysial joint	Osteophytes
	Ganglion
	Tumor
	Rheumatoid arthritis
	Gout
	Ankylosing spondylitis
	Fracture
Vertebral body	Tumor
	Paget's disease
	Fracture
	Osteomyelitis
	Hydatid
	Hyperparathyroidism
Meninges	Cysts
	Meningioma
	Dermoid cyst
	Epidermoid cyst
	Epidural abscess
	Epidural hematoma
Blood vessels	Angioma
	Arteritis
Nerve sheath	Neurofibroma
	Schwannoma
Nerve	Neuroblastoma
	Ganglioneuroma

activity in afferent fibers; but that activity occurs in Aβ fibers as well as C fibers.[2,3] Therefore, the activity is something more than simply nociceptive. This finding underlies and underscores the particular nature of radicular pain. It is shooting, stabbing, or electric in nature, traveling distally into the affected limb, which is consistent with a massive discharge from multiple affected axons. It is commonly associated with paresthesiae; which is consistent with Aβ fibers being included in the discharge.

As opposed to compression, there are growing contentions that cervical radicular pain may be caused by inflammation of the cervical nerve roots. This mechanism might be applicable to radicular pain caused by disc protrusions, because inflammatory exudates have now been isolated from cervical disc material.[4,5] However, inflammation cannot be invoked as the mechanism of radicular pain caused by noninflammatory lesions such as tumors, cysts, and osteophytes. For these conditions, compression of the dorsal root ganglion is the only mechanism for which there is experimental evidence.

However, none of these considerations bear on the causes and mechanisms of neck pain. Whatever its cause, and whatever its mechanism, cervical radicular pain is perceived in the upper limb. This characteristic has been clearly shown in experiments in which cervical spinal nerves have been deliberately provoked with needles.[6] The subjects report pain spreading throughout the length of the upper limb. But unlike the sensory loss of cervical radiculopathy, the pattern of cervical radicular pain is not dermatomal. Radicular pain is perceived deeply, through the shoulder girdle and into the upper limb proper. Radicular pain from C5 tends to remain in the arm, but pain from C6, C7, and C8 extends into the forearm and hand. These patterns of distribution indicate that the pain is not restricted to cutaneous afferents. It involves afferents from deep tissues as well, such as muscles and joints. Because the segmental innervation of deep tissues is not the same as that of skin, radicular pain cannot be, and is not, dermatomal in distribution. In particular, muscles of the shoulder girdle are innervated by C6 and C7, well away from the dermatomes of these nerves. If anything, the segmental innervation of muscles is a better guide to the distribution of radicular pain than are the dermatomes. Dermatomes are nonetheless relevant for the distribution of the neurologic signs of radiculopathy, but this has nothing to do with the distribution of pain.

NECK PAIN

By definition, neck pain is pain perceived as arising in a region bounded superiorly by the superior nuchal line, laterally by the lateral margins of the neck, and inferiorly by an imaginary transverse line through the T1 spinous process.[7] This definition does not presuppose, nor does it imply, that the cause of pain lies within this area. It defines neck pain simply by where the patient feels the pain. An objective of clinical practice is to determine exactly the source and cause of this pain, and then to implement measures to stop it.

Sources of Neck Pain

The notion of source of pain is different from that of the cause of pain. A source is defined in anatomic terms, and pertains to the site from which nociception is generated, without reference to its actual cause.

Potential sources

For a structure to be a potential source of pain it must be innervated. In this regard, there is abundant information concerning the cervical spine.

The posterior neck muscles and the cervical zygapophysial joints are innervated by the cervical dorsal rami.[8] The lateral atlantoaxial joint is innervated by the C2 ventral ramus,[9] and the atlantooccipital joint is supplied by the C1 ventral ramus.[9] The median atlantoaxial joint and its ligaments are supplied by the sinuvertebral nerves of C1, C2, and C3.[10] These nerves also supply the dura mater of the cervical spinal cord.[10,11] The innervation of the prevertebral and lateral muscles of the neck has not been studied in modern times, but textbooks of anatomy affirm that these are supplied by branches of the cervical ventral rami.[12]

The cervical intervertebral discs receive an innervation from multiple sources. Posteriorly, they receive branches from a posterior vertebral plexus that lies on the floor of the vertebral canal, and which is formed by the cervical sinuvertebral nerves.[13–15] Anteriorly, they receive branches from an anterior vertebral plexus that is formed by the cervical sympathetic trunks.[13] Laterally, they receive branches from the vertebral nerve.[14]

The vertebral nerve is formed by branches of the cervical gray rami communicantes, and accompanies the vertebral artery.[16] In addition to giving rise to the sinuvertebral nerves, the vertebral nerve provides a somatic (sensory) innervation to the vertebral artery.[17]

On the grounds that they are innervated, all of the muscles, synovial joints, and intervertebral discs of the neck are potential sources of neck pain, along with the cervical dura mater and the vertebral artery. However, innervation is insufficient grounds alone to credit that these structures are sources of neck pain. For a structure to be credited as a potential source, physiologic evidence of its potential is required.

In that regard, sources of neck pain have been studied in 2 ways. In normal volunteers, various structures have been studied experimentally to determine if possibly they can, and therefore could, produce neck pain. In patients suffering from neck pain, the same sites have been anesthetized to determine if doing so relieves the pain.

Normal volunteers

Classic experiments involved the noxious stimulation of posterior midline structures with injections of hypertonic saline.[18–20] These experiments showed that such stimulation produces not only local neck pain but also somatic referred pain. The distribution of referred pain related to the segment stimulated. Accordingly, stimulation of upper cervical segments produced referred pain into the head; stimulation of lower cervical segments produced referred pain into the shoulder girdle and upper limb.

These experiments were important because they showed the phenomenon of somatic referred pain. They showed that disorders of the cervical spine could produce headache, as well as pain in the upper limb. In both instances the mechanism did not involve irritation of nerve roots. The mechanism involves convergence. Nociceptive afferents from the cervical spine converge with afferents from distal sites, on second-order neurons in the spinal cord. Under these conditions, spinal pain can be perceived as also arising from those distal sites.

It has been shown that noxious stimulation of the cervical zygapophysial joints causes neck pain and referred pain. The observations have been corroborated using a variety of stimuli. One series of experiments used a mechanical stimulus, in the form of an injection of contrast medium, to distend the target joint.[21,22] Another used the same mechanical stimulus but also used electrical stimulation of the nerves that innervated the target joint.[23] Both approaches found the same outcomes.

Pain from the cervical zygapophysial joints tends to follow relatively constant and recognizable patterns (**Fig. 1**). From the C2-3 level it is referred rostrally to the head. From C3-4 and C4-5 it is located over the posterior neck. From C5-6 it spreads

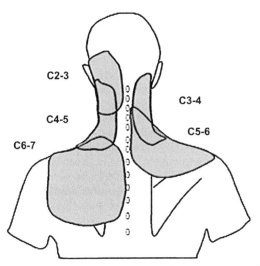

Fig. 1. The distribution of pain in normal volunteers after stimulation of the zygapophysial joints indicated. (*From* Cooper G, Bailey B, Bogduk N. Cervical zygapophysial joint pain maps. Pain Med 2007;8:344–53; with permission.)

over the supraspinous fossa of the scapula. From C6-7 it spreads further caudally over the scapula.

Essentially similar patterns of pain have been produced by mechanical stimulation of cervical intervertebral discs.[24–26] This fact underscores the rule that it is not the structure that determines the pattern of pain stemming from it, but its nerve supply. Thus, any structure innervated by the same cervical segmental nerves has the same distribution of pain. This observation means that, clinically, discogenic pain cannot be distinguished from zygapophysial joint pain, but the distribution of pain serves as a reasonable guide to the most likely segmental location of its source.

In principle, this rule would also apply to neck muscles. Pain from muscles innervated by a particular segment should be perceived in the same location as pain from articular structures innervated by the same segment. However, there have been no systematic studies of neck pain from muscles in normal volunteers. The only study involving neck muscles showed that stimulation of upper cervical muscles could produce pain in the head.[27]

Other structures that have been shown to be able to produce neck pain and headache in normal volunteers are the atlantooccipital and the lateral atlantoaxial joints.[28] Pain from these structures does not occur in a unique distribution. Along with the C2-3 joints, these structures all produce pain in the suboccipital region.

Clinical studies

As a complement to the studies in normal volunteers, clinical studies have provided evidence of the sources of pain in patients with neck pain. They involved either the anaesthetization or the provocation of pain.

Several studies have shown that anesthetizing the cervical zygapophysial joints can relieve neck pain.[29–34] The most powerful of these used controlled, diagnostic blocks: either comparative local anesthetic blocks, or placebo-controlled blocks, each on a double-blind basis.

One such study examined the distribution of pain that was relieved by controlled diagnostic blocks of the zygapophysial joints at various segments, or of the lateral atlantoaxial joint.[34] It found that, although patients conformed in general terms to the pain maps developed in normal volunteers (see **Fig. 1**), they differed greatly with respect to the patterns of distribution. Whereas some patients might suffer narrow areas of pain, others might suffer wider areas; and whereas some patients might suffer pain in longer (ie, taller) distributions, in others the distribution might be shorter. Consequently, no single pattern of distribution was characteristic of pain from a given segment, but certain rules emerged (**Fig. 2**).

Pain from C1-2 and pain from C2-3 are similar in distribution. Both tend to center over the suboccipital region and radiate, to various extents, to the occiput, auricular region, vertex of the head, forehead, and orbit. In the head, pain from C1-2 tends to occur higher than pain from C2-3, in the vertex rather than in the forehead and temple.

Pain from C3-4 resembles that from C2-3 but tends to radiate more caudally into the neck. Pain from C4-5 tends to nestle into the angle between the lower end of the neck and the top of the shoulder girdle.

Pain from C5-6 and from C6-7 both encompass the lower neck and the shoulder girdle. Pain from C5-6 tends to radiate more laterally, over the deltoid region and into the arm. Pain from C6-7 tends to radiate more medially, over the medial scapula.

Other studies have used provocation discography to implicate the cervical intervertebral discs as sources of neck pain.[25,26,35] However, discography is a capricious test. Even if performed carefully, with attention to testing control levels, it can be subject to false-positive responses.[35] Moreover, in patients with neck pain, it is uncommon to find a single disc that seems to be painful. If all cervical discs are tested, 2, 3, or more can be found to be painful. Under those conditions, it is difficult to determine whether various discs are truly multiple, simultaneous sources of neck pain or whether the patient is simply expressing hyperalgesia. Nevertheless, the clinical data are consistent with observations in normal volunteers that the cervical discs are possible sources of neck pain.

Several studies have reported that the C2-3 zygapophysial joint can be the source of pain in many patients with headache.[35–37] Anesthetizing the joint completely abolishes

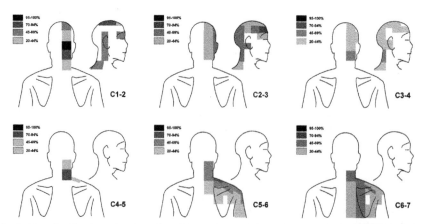

Fig. 2. The distribution of pain relieved in patients with neck pain, after anesthetization of the synovial joints indicated, using controlled diagnostic blocks. The density of shading is proportional to the number of patients whose pain extended into the area indicated. (*From* Cooper G, Bailey B, Bogduk N. Cervical zygapophysial joint pain maps. Pain Med 2007;8:344–53; with permission.)

the headache in these patients. Other studies have reported the same results after anesthetization of the lateral atlantoaxial joints.[35,38–40]

Other tissues, such as the posterior neck muscles, the cervical dura mater, the median atlantoaxial joint and its ligaments, and the vertebral artery are potential sources of neck pain, because they are all innervated, but they have not been subjected to study either in normal volunteers or in patients. That they could be sources of pain is a credible proposition, but formal evidence is lacking.

Implications

The experimental data, from normal volunteers and from patients, indicate the synovial joints and intervertebral discs of the neck are potential sources of neck pain. Other tissues such as muscles, ligaments, the dura mater, and the vertebral artery, are in theory potential sources of pain. For a structure to be promoted from a potential to an actual source of pain, it needs to be affected by a disorder capable of causing pain.

Causes of Neck Pain

Hearsay and imaging have been the traditional basis for listing causes of neck pain. Particular conditions have been regarded as a cause of neck pain simply because someone once said they were, or because they can be seen on a radiograph. Both are weak arguments subject to large errors.

Hearsay allows any conjecture to be raised as a possible cause of neck pain, but when these are listed in textbooks they tend to assume an undeserved status of veracity. Once a condition is listed, consumers tend to accept that it is a possible cause of neck pain, and proponents are excused the responsibility of providing corroborating evidence.

The necessary evidence is some objective test that confirms the presence of the condition, and which can be used to show both that the condition occurs in patients with neck pain and that it does not occur in patients without neck pain. For some conditions, the objective test may be a radiograph, but other conditions are not visible on radiographs. For these latter conditions some other from of evidence is required.

It transpires that for most entities, an objective test is not available or has not been applied. Consequently, there is no evidence that these conditions cause neck pain; they are no more than conjectures. In some instances, applying objective tests has resulted in certain, sometimes hallowed, entities being refuted as causes of neck pain.

Typical of lists of purported causes of neck pain are those published in leading textbooks of rheumatology (**Table 2**). The lists are not identical, but there is considerable agreement about several conditions.

These purported causes of neck pain can be grouped in 3 ways: according to clinical significance into serious or nonthreatening conditions; into common and uncommon conditions; and into valid and not valid causes.

Serious but rare conditions are the neoplasms and infections. No-one seriously doubts the legitimacy of such conditions as causes of neck pain because, by and large, they can be diagnosed by medical imaging and by biopsy, if required. However, they are rare. In population studies of patients presenting with neck pain, unsuspected tumors and infections have never been disclosed.[44,45] Given the size of these studies, calculation of 95% confidence intervals reveals that serious conditions account for less than 0.4% of cases of neck pain.

Overlooked by contemporary textbooks is the importance of vascular disorders in the diagnosis of neck pain. Although headache is the most common presenting feature of internal carotid artery dissection, neck pain has been the sole presenting feature in some 6% of cases.[46,47] In 17% of patients headache may occur in

Table 2
Causes of neck pain as listed in 3 major textbooks of rheumatology, with concordance between sources indicated

Causes	Nakano[41]	Hardin and Halla[42]	Binder[43]
Serious but Rare			
Vertebral tumors	++	++	++
Discitis	++	++	—
Septic arthritis	++	++	—
Osteomyelitis	++	++	++
Meningitis	++	++	—
Valid but Rare or Unusual			
Rheumatoid arthritis	++	++	++
Ankylosing spondylitis	++	++	—
Crystal arthropathies including gout	++	++	++
Polymyalgia rheumatica	—	++	++
Longus colli tendonitis	—	++	—
Fractures	—	++	—
Miscellaneous			
Torticollis	++	++	++
Detectable but of Questionable Validity			
Diffuse idiopathic skeletal hyperostosis	++	++	++
Ossification of the posterior longitudinal ligament	—	—	++
Paget's disease	++	++	++
Spondylosis/degenerative disease	++	++	++
Osteoarthritis	++	—	—
Synovial cyst	—	++	—
Neurologic			
Thoracic outlet syndrome	++	++	++
Spinal cord tumors	++	—	—
Nerve injuries	++	—	—
Myelopathy	—	—	++
Radiculopathy	—	—	++
Spurious or Vague			
Soft-tissue injuries	—	++	—
Whiplash	—	—	++
Cervical strain	++	—	—
Psychogenic	—	—	++
Postural disorders	++	—	++
Fibrositis, myofascial pain	++	++	++
Hyoid bone syndrome	—	++	—
Sternocleidomastoid tendonitis	++	—	—
Fibromyalgia	—	++	—

combination with neck pain.[47] Neck pain has been the initial presenting feature in 50% to 90% of patients with vertebral artery dissection, but is usually also accompanied by headache, typically in the occipital region although not exclusively so.[46,48] Although the typical features of dissecting aneurysms of the aorta are chest pain and cardiovascular distress, neck pain has been reported as the presenting feature in some 6% of cases.[49,50] However, all of these vascular conditions are unlikely to be causes of persistent neck pain, because in due course they all develop additional clinical features, sometimes rapidly, that implicate a vascular disorder.

Less serious conditions are the inflammatory arthropathies. The validity of these conditions as a cause of neck pain is not questioned, because the condition can be detected by imaging, and these conditions are accepted, recognized causes of joint pain when they affect the joints of the appendicular skeleton. However, these conditions typically affect the neck in patients with evidence of systemic distribution of arthropathy. They are rare causes of neck pain alone.

Polymyalgia rheumatica is a valid entity, but it should not be listed as a cause of neck pain. It is a condition that may involve the neck but, by definition, it is a systemic disorder that affects other regions of the body as well. It does not present with isolated neck pain. Similar comments and deletions apply to fibromyalgia. Regardless of whether one accepts that fibromyalgia is a valid entity or not, it is, by definition, a widespread disorder, and not one that enters the differential diagnosis of neck pain as an isolated symptom.

Longus colli tendonitis is a misnomer for a condition better known as retropharyngeal tendinitis,[51-58] because the condition involves more than just the tendons of the prevertebral muscles. It involves inflammation and edema of the upper portions of the longus colli (not just its tendons), from the level of C1 to C4 and even to C6.[51-53] It is a rare condition, but can be diagnosed by plain radiography, and most accurately by magnetic resonance imaging (MRI).[53]

Fractures are an accepted cause of pain, although not all fractures are necessarily painful. As causes of neck pain, however, fractures are rare or unusual. Like tumors, unsuspected fractures proved to have zero prevalence in large population surveys,[44,45] which places their prevalence at less than 0.4%. Even amongst patients presenting to emergency rooms, with suspected or possible cervical trauma, fractures are uncommon.[59-67] A prevalence figure of 3.5% ($\pm$ 0.5%) is representative.

Synovial cyst is a spurious cause of neck pain. There are no reports of this condition causing neck pain. When symptomatic, these cysts cause radiculopathy or radicular pain.[68-70] Accordingly, they do not constitute a differential diagnosis of neck pain.

Torticollis is a clinical syndrome; it is not a specific cause of neck pain. It is characterized by fixed rotation of the head and cervical spine. The neck may or may not be painful, but the presentation does not define the cause, or even the source, of pain. In adults, known causes include basal ganglion disorders, subluxation of the lateral atlantoaxial joint,[71-75] and epidural abscess.[76] Speculative causes include subluxations of the zygapophysial joints and extrapment of their meniscoids.[77]

Several listed conditions constitute detectable disorders but questionable sources of neck pain. Diffuse idiopathic skeletal hyperostosis can be vividly shown on radiographs of affected regions of the spine, but it is often asymptomatic.[42,43] When symptomatic it causes stiffness and dysphagia, rather than neck pain.[42,43] Similarly, ossification of the posterior longitudinal ligament can be asymptomatic.[42,43] Rather than neck pain, this condition is more likely to present with myelopathy.[42,43]

Paget's disease is, as a general rule, an accepted cause of pain in the body regions affected. Technically, therefore, it is an acceptable cause of neck pain if detected in the cervical spine. However, 1 large survey found that Paget's disease is often painless, and that patients with cervical spine involvement had no pain complaints referable to that region.[78] This finding gives cause to doubt that Paget's disease is ever a cause of neck pain. When diagnosed radiologically, Paget's disease in the cervical spine may be no more than an incidental finding.

Spondylosis and osteoarthritis are perhaps the most commonly applied diagnoses in patients with neck pain with demonstrable changes on radiographs. However, neither diagnosis is valid. The radiographic features of cervical spondylosis occur with increasing frequency with increasing age in asymptomatic individuals.[79,80] This finding indicates that these features are age-related changes. Most commonly they affect the C5-6 and C6-7 segments. However, these changes are weakly, if at all, associated with pain. In some studies, cervical spondylosis occurs somewhat more commonly in symptomatic individuals than in asymptomatic individuals,[44,81] but the odds ratios for disc degeneration or osteoarthrosis as predictors of neck pain are only 1.1 and 0.97, respectively, for women and 1.7 and 1.8 for men.[81] In other studies, the prevalence of disc degeneration, at individual segments of the neck, is not significantly different between symptomatic patients and asymptomatic controls.[82] Uncovertebral osteophytes and osteoarthrosis were found to be less prevalent in symptomatic individuals.[82] Consequently, finding spondylosis or osteoarthritis on a radiograph does not constitute making a diagnosis or finding the source of pain.

The various neurologic conditions listed in **Table 2** are, by definition, not causes of neck pain. They cause symptoms, not in the neck, but in the upper limb. Furthermore, they cause loss of neurologic function rather than pain.

The remaining, listed causes of neck pain are little more than spurious labels. Yet it is these labels that are so often applied to most patients with neck pain.

Soft-tissue injury means nothing more than that something has been injured but there has not been a fracture. Whiplash describes the possible cause of the pain but not its cause or its source. Cervical strain is an ambiguous term that implies no more than that something went wrong with the neck to produce pain.

Psychogenic pain is a dated, but often abused, term. It is not admitted by the *Diagnostic and Statistical Manual of Mental Disorders, Fourth Edition*.[83] Unless an alternative, specific psychiatric diagnosis is proffered, psychogenic pain is a euphemism for "I don't know what's wrong" or for malingering.

Although sometimes invoked as a diagnosis, postural disorders may be secondary to neck pain. There is no evidence that some sort of habitual abnormal posture causes pain. Such prospective, longitudinal, long-term data as are available indicate that abnormal posture does not lead to a greater incidence of pain.[84]

Although commonly held to be a cause of neck pain, myofascial disorders fail on several counts. The cardinal diagnostic feature for myofascial pain is the detection of a trigger point. However, there is no evidence that examiners can reliably detect trigger points in the neck, but the classic trigger points of the neck do not satisfy the prescribed criteria for a trigger point, to the extent that they are exempt from doing so.[85] The features of cervical trigger points seem better to describe a tender, underlying zygapophysial joint, and the pain associated with those trigger points is identical in distribution to the pain that would arise from the underlying joint.[86]

Hyoid bone syndrome is a poorly studied condition. Its features are said to be tenderness over the greater cornu of the hyoid bone. Hyoid syndrome might be included in the differential diagnosis of anterior neck pain, but it cannot be confused with posterior neck pain. The diagnostic criterion is said to be relief of pain on anesthetizing the cornu,[87] but no studies have tested this criterion under controlled conditions.

Beyond being listed recurrently in textbooks, there is little literature on sternocleidomastoid tendonitis. The cardinal diagnostic feature seems to be tenderness over the tendons of the muscle, but this has not been distinguished from random hyperalgesia in patients with neck pain.

Implications

A sober review of the purported causes of neck pain reveals that the most readily diagnosed and serious conditions are rare, and do not account for most cases. Meanwhile, the most commonly applied diagnoses lack validity. Either they have been disproved by epidemiologic studies or they have defied testing. Other entities are descriptive terms but not proper diagnoses. For common, uncomplicated neck pain there are no data on its cause.

DISCUSSION

For the management of acute neck pain, there is little need for a knowledge of the sources, causes, or mechanisms of pain. Tumors and infections are rare, and should be associated with alerting clues from the patient's history. Otherwise, the natural history of acute neck pain is such that most cases recover regardless, and even despite treatment. For the treatment of acute neck pain after whiplash, 2 studies have shown that no more sophisticated intervention is required than a schedule of home exercises.[88,89,90] Another study has shown that advice to resume normal activities is all that is required.[91]

Nevertheless, despite the favorable natural history of acute neck pain, a proportion of patients develop chronic neck pain. The magnitude of that proportion is not certain but 10% to 30% seems a reasonable estimate. For those patients, a knowledge of the sources, and possible causes, of pain becomes pertinent, because it can determine what measures are taken to investigate it and to treat it.

At present, the only valid data pertain to cervical zygapophysial joint pain. Several studies have now shown that these joints are a common source of chronic neck pain.[30-33] Three studies have indicated that zygapophysial joint pain is the single most common basis for chronic neck pain after whiplash. It accounts for at least 50% of cases,[31,32] and up to 80% of victims of high-speed collisions.[92] Comparable studies in patients with no history of whiplash have been undertaken.

However, the cause of zygapophysial joint pain is not known. Postmortem studies implicate subchondral fractures and contusions of the intra-articular meniscoids.[93-95] Such lesions are consistent with the biomechanics of whiplash,[96] but they have defied detection in vivo. Contemporary techniques of medical imaging do not have the resolution to identify these lesions. High-resolution computed tomography scanning might be able to identify subchondral fractures, if the joints were subjected to serial 1-mm sections; but no-one has undertaken such studies. Reports of fractures to the zygapophysial joints have been limited to occasional case studies or small case series.[97-101]

Biomechanics studies predict that anterior tears of the annulus fibrosus could also be a lesion of whiplash,[96] but these too have defied detection in vivo. Although 1 MRI study reported a rim lesion in a cervical disc in a patient with a whiplash-associated disorder,[102] subsequent studies have failed to corroborate this finding.[103-108]

More vexatious is providing an explanation for chronic neck pain not caused by trauma. This form of neck pain cannot be attributed to spondylosis. Yet even if that label were accepted it does not provide a mechanism for the pain or its source. There is no known mechanism whereby an aging disc should spontaneously become painful.

Perhaps attractive is the proposition that osteoarthritis of the zygapophysial joint is the basis for atraumatic neck pain. However, this diagnosis cannot be made from radiographic findings. It requires some other objective test, such as performing controlled, diagnostic blocks of the suspected, painful joint. Such studies have yet to be conducted.

Similarly, for any other purported cause of neck pain, appropriate studies have yet to be conducted. We have yet to see compelling data, from controlled studies, that show that muscles, ligaments, or other cervical structures are the source of chronic neck pain.

REFERENCES

1. Bogduk N. Medical management of acute cervical radicular pain. An evidence-based approach. Newcastle (UK): Newcastle Bone and Joint Institute; 1999.
2. Howe JF. A neurophysiological basis for the radicular pain of nerve root compression. In: Bonica JJ, Liebeskind JC, Albe-Fessard DG, editors, Advances in pain research and therapy, vol. 3. New York: Raven Press; 1979. p. 647–57.
3. Howe JF, Loeser JD, Calvin WH. Mechanosensitivity of dorsal root ganglia and chronically injured axons: a physiological basis for the radicular pain of nerve root compression. Pain 1977;3:25–41.
4. Kang JD, Georgescu HI, McIntyre-Larkin L, et al. Herniated cervical interverte-bral discs spontaneously produce matrix metalloproteinases, nitric oxide, interleukin-6 and prostaglandin E_2. Spine 1995;22:2373–8.
5. Furusawa N, Baba H, Miyoshi N, et al. Herniation of cervical intervertebral disc. Immunohistochemical examination and measurement of nitric oxide production. Spine 2001;26:1110–6.
6. Slipman CW, Plastaras CT, Palmitier RA, et al. Symptom provocation of fluoro-scopically guided cervical nerve root stimulation: are dynatomal maps identical to dermatomal maps? Spine 1998;23:2235–42.
7. Merskey H, Bogduk N, editors. Classification of chronic pain. Descriptions of chronic pain syndromes and definition of pain terms. 2nd edition. Seattle (WA): IASP Press; 1994. p. 103–11.
8. Bogduk N. The clinical anatomy of the cervical dorsal rami. Spine 1982;7: 319–30.
9. Lazorthes G, Gaubert J. L'innervation des articulations interapophysaire verte-brales. Comptes Rendues de l'Association des Anatomistes 1956;43:488–94 [in French].
10. Kimmel DL. Innervation of the spinal dura mater and dura mater of the posterior cranial fossa. Neurology 1960;10:800–9.
11. Groen GJ, Baljet B, Drukker J. The innervation of the spinal dura mater: anatomy and clinical implications. Acta Neurochir 1988;92:39–46.
12. Williams PL, editor. Gray's anatomy. 38th edition. Edinburgh (UK): Churchill Livingstone; 1995. p. 808.
13. Groen GJ, Baljet B, Drukker J. Nerves and nerve plexuses of the human verte-bral column. Am J Anat 1990;188:282–96.
14. Bogduk N, Windsor M, Inglis A. The innervation of the cervical intervertebral discs. Spine 1988;13:2–8.
15. Mendel T, Wink CS, Zimny ML. Neural elements in human cervical intervertebral discs. Spine 1992;17:132–5.
16. Bogduk N, Lambert G, Duckworth JW. The anatomy and physiology of the verte-bral nerve in relation to cervical migraine. Cephalalgia 1981;1:11–24.
17. Kimmel DL. The cervical sympathetic rami and the vertebral plexus in the human foetus. J Comp Neurol 1959;112:141–61.

18. Campbell DG, Parsons CM. Referred head pain and its concomitants. J Nerv Ment Dis 1944;99:544–51.
19. Kellgren JH. On the distribution of pain arising from deep somatic structures with charts of segmental pain areas. Clin Sci 1939;4:35–46.
20. Feinstein B, Langton JB, Jameson RM, et al. Experiments on referred pain from deep somatic tissues. J Bone Joint Surg Am 1954;36:981–97.
21. Dwyer A, Aprill C, Bogduk N. Cervical zygapophysial joint pain patterns I: a study in normal volunteers. Spine 1990;15:453–7.
22. Aprill C, Dwyer A, Bogduk N. Cervical zygapophyseal joint pain patterns II: a clinical evaluation. Spine 1990;15:458–61.
23. Fukui S, Ohseto K, Shiotani M, et al. Referred pain distribution of the cervical zygapophyseal joints and cervical dorsal rami. Pain 1996;68:79–83.
24. Cloward RB. Cervical diskography. A contribution to the aetiology and mechanism of neck, shoulder and arm pain. Ann Surg 1959;130:1052–64.
25. Schellhas KP, Smith MD, Gundry CR, et al. Cervical discogenic pain: prospective correlation of magnetic resonance imaging and discography in asymptomatic subjects and pain sufferers. Spine 1996;21:300–12.
26. Grubb SA, Kelly CK. Cervical discography: clinical implications from 12 years of experience. Spine 2000;25:1382–9.
27. Cyriax J. Rheumatic headache. BMJ 1938;2:1367–8.
28. Dreyfuss P, Michaelsen M, Fletcher D. Atlanto-occipital and lateral atlanto-axial joint pain patterns. Spine 1994;19:1125–31.
29. Bogduk N, Marsland A. The cervical zygapophysial joints as a source of neck pain. Spine 1988;13:610–7.
30. Aprill C, Bogduk N. The prevalence of cervical zygapophyseal joint pain: a first approximation. Spine 1992;17:744–7.
31. Barnsley L, Lord SM, Wallis BJ, et al. The prevalence of chronic cervical zygapophysial joint pain after whiplash. Spine 1995;20:20–6.
32. Lord S, Barnsley L, Wallis BJ, et al. Chronic cervical zygapophysial joint pain after whiplash: a placebo-controlled prevalence study. Spine 1996;21:1737–45.
33. Speldewinde GC, Bashford GM, Davidson IR. Diagnostic cervical zygapophysial joint blocks for chronic cervical pain. Med J Aust 2001;174:174–6.
34. Cooper G, Bailey B, Bogduk N. Cervical zygapophysial joint pain maps. Pain Med 2007;8:344–53.
35. Bogduk N, Aprill C. On the nature of neck pain, discography and cervical zygapophysial joint pain. Pain 1993;54:213–7.
36. Bogduk N, Marsland A. On the concept of third occipital headache. J Neurol Neurosurg Psychiatry 1986;49:775–80.
37. Lord S, Barnsley L, Wallis B, et al. Third occipital headache: a prevalence study. J Neurol Neurosurg Psychiatry 1994;57:1187–90.
38. Ehni G, Benner B. Occipital neuralgia and the C1-2 arthrosis syndrome. J Neurosurg 1984;61:961–5.
39. Busch E, Wilson PR. Atlanto-occipital and atlanto-axial injections in the treatment of headache and neck pain. Reg Anesth 1989;14(Suppl 2):45.
40. Aprill C, Axinn MJ, Bogduk N. Occipital headaches stemming from the lateral atlanto-axial (C1-2) joint. Cephalalgia 2002;22:15–22.
41. Nakano KK. Neck pain. In: Ruddy S, Harris ED, Sledge CB, editors. Kelley's textbook of rheumatology. 6th edition. Philadelphia: WB Saunders; 2001. p. 457–74.
42. Hardin JG, Halla JT. Cervical spine syndromes. In: Koopman WJ, editor. Arthritis and allied conditions. A textbook of rheumatology. 14th edition. Philadelphia: Lippincott Williams & Wilkins; 2001. p. 2009–18.

43. Binder A. Cervical pain syndromes. In: Maddison PJ, Isenberg DA, Woo P, et al, editors. Oxford textbook of rheumatology. Oxford (UK): Oxford University Press; 1993. p. 1060–70.
44. Heller CA, Stanley P, Lewis-Jones B, et al. Value of x ray examinations of the cervical spine. BMJ 1983;287:1276–8.
45. Johnson MJ, Lucas GL. Value of cervical spine radiographs as a screening tool. Clin Orthop 1997;340:102–8.
46. Silbert PL, Makri B, Schievink WI. Headache and neck pain in spontaneous internal carotid and vertebral artery dissections. Neurology 1995;45: 1517–22.
47. Biousse V, D'Anglejan-Chatillon J, Massiou H, et al. Head pain in non-traumatic carotid artery dissection: a series of 65 patients. Cephalalgia 1994;14:33–6.
48. Sturzenegger M. Headache and neck pain: the warning symptoms of vertebral artery dissection. Headache 1994;34:187–93.
49. Garrard P, Barnes D. Aortic dissection presenting as a neurological emergency. J R Soc Med 1996;89:271–2.
50. Hirst AE, Johns VJ, Kime FW. Dissecting aneurysm of the aorta: a review of 505 cases. Medicine 1958;37:217–75.
51. Fahlgren H. Retropharyngeal tendonitis. Cephalalgia 1986;6:169–74.
52. Sarkozi J, Fam AG. Acute calcific retropharyngeal tendonitis: an unusual cause of neck pain. Arthritis Rheum 1984;27:708–10.
53. Ekbom K, Torhall J, Annell K, et al. Magnetic resonance image in retropharyngeal tendonitis. Cephalalgia 1994;14:266–9.
54. Karasick D, Karasick S. Calcific retropharyngeal tendonitis. Skeletal Radiol 1981;7:203–5.
55. Hartley J. Acute cervical pain associated with retropharyngeal calcium deposit. J Bone Joint Surg Am 1964;46:1753–4.
56. Bernstein SA. Acute cervical pain associated with soft-tissue calcium deposition anterior to the interspace of the first and second cervical vertebrae. J Bone Joint Surg Am 1975;57:426–8.
57. Newmark H, Forrester DM, Brown JC, et al. Calcific tendonitis of the neck. Radiology 1978;128:355–8.
58. Newmark H, Zee CS, Frankel P, et al. Chronic calcific tendonitis of the neck. Skeletal Radiol 1981;7:207–8 Am J Surg 1987.
59. Fischer RP. Cervical radiographic evaluation of alert patients following blunt trauma. Ann Emerg Med 1984;13:905–7.
60. Jacobs LM, Schwartz R. Prospective analysis of acute cervical spine injury: a methodology to predict injury. Ann Emerg Med 1986;15:44–9.
61. Mace SE. Emergency evaluation of cervical spine injuries: CT versus plain radiographs. Ann Emerg Med 1985;14:973–5.
62. Roberge RJ, Wears RC, Kelly M, et al. Selective application of cervical spine radiography in alert victims of blunt trauma: a prospective study. J Trauma 1988;28:784–8.
63. McNamara RM. Post-traumatic neck pain: a prospective and follow-up study. Ann Emerg Med 1988;17;906–11.
64. Kreipke DL, Gillespie KR, McCarthy MC, et al. Reliability of indications for cervical spine films in trauma patients. J Trauma 1989;29:1438–9.
65. Hoffman JR, Schriger DL, Mower W, et al. Low-risk criteria for cervical-spine radiography in blunt trauma: a prospective study. Ann Emerg Med 1992;21: 1454–60.

66. Gerrelts BD, Petersen EU, Mabry J, et al. Delayed diagnosis of cervical spine injuries. J Trauma 1991;31:1622–6.
67. Bachulis BL, Long WB, Hynes GD, et al. Clinical indications for cervical spine radiographs in the traumatized patient. Am J Surg 1987;153:473–7.
68. Takano Y, Homma T, Okumura H, et al. Ganglion cyst occurring in the ligamentum flavum of the cervical spine. Case report. Spine 1992;17:1531–3.
69. Lunardi P, Acqui M, Ricci G, et al. Cervical synovial cysts: case report and review of the literature. Eur Spine J 1999;8:232–7.
70. Shima Y, Rothman SLG, Yasura K, et al. Degenerative intraspinal cyst of the cervical spine. Case report and literature review. Spine 2002;27:E18–22.
71. Wortzman G, Dewar FP. Rotatory fixation of the atlantoaxial joint: rotational atlantoaxial subluxation. Radiology 1968;90:479–87.
72. Jayakrishnan VK, Teasdale E. Torticollis due to atlanto-axial rotatory fixation following general anaesthesia. Br J Neurosurg 2000;14:583–5.
73. Wise JJ, Cheney R, Fischgrund J. Traumatic bilateral rotatory dislocation of the atlanto-axial joints: a case report and review of the literature. J Spinal Disord 1997;10:451–3.
74. Fielding JW, Hawkins RJ. Atlanto-axial rotatory fixation (fixed rotatory subluxation of the atlanto-axial joint). J Bone Joint Surg Am 1977;59:37–44.
75. Van Holsbeeck EM, Mackay NN. Diagnosis of acute atlanto-axial rotatory fixation. J Bone Joint Surg Br 1989;71:90–1.
76. McKnight P, Friedman J. Torticollis due to cervical epidural abscess and osteomyelitis. Neurology 1992;42:696–7.
77. Mercer S, Bogduk N. Intra-articular inclusions of the cervical synovial joints. Br J Rheumatol 1993;32:705–10.
78. Harinck HI, Buvoet OL, Vellenga CJ, et al. Relation between signs and symptoms in Paget's disease of bone. Q J Med 1986;58:133–51.
79. Gore DR, Sepic SB, Gardner GM. Roentgenographic findings of the cervical spine in asymptomatic people. Spine 1986;1:521–4.
80. Elias F. Roentgen findings in the asymptomatic cervical spine. N Y State J Med 1958;58:3300–3.
81. Van der Donk J, Schouten JS, Passchier J, et al. The associations of neck pain with radiological abnormalities of the cervical spine and personality traits in a general population. J Rheumatol 1991;18:1884–9.
82. Fridenberg ZB, Miller WT. Degenerative disc disease of the cervical spine. A comparative study of asymptomatic and symptomatic patients. J Bone Joint Surg Am 1963;45:1171–8.
83. DSM-IV. Diagnostic and statistical manual of mental disorders. 4th edition. Washington, DC: American Psychiatric Association; 1994. p. 683.
84. Dieck GS, Kelsey JL, Goel VK, et al. An epidemiologic study of the relationship between postural asymmetry in the teen years and subsequent back and neck pain. Spine 1985;10:872–7.
85. Travell JG, Simons DG. Myofascial pain and dysfunction. The trigger point manual. Baltimore (MD): Williams & Wilkins; 1993. p. 312.
86. Bogduk N, Simons DG. Neck pain: joint pain or trigger points. In: Vaeroy H, Merskey H, editors. Progress in fibromyalgia and myofascial pain. Amsterdam: Elsevier; 1993. p. 267–73.
87. Robinson PJ, Davis JP, Fraser JG. The hyoid syndrome: a pain in the neck. J Laryngol Otol 1994;108:855–8.
88. McKinney LA. Early mobilisation and outcomes in acute sprains of the neck. BMJ 1989;299:1006–8.

89. McKinney LA, Dornan JO, Ryan M. The role of physiotherapy in the management of acute neck sprains following road-traffic accidents. Arch Emerg Med 1989;6:27–33.

90. Rosenfeld M, Gunnarsson R, Borenstein P. Early intervention in whiplash-associated disorders. A comparison of two treatment protocols. Spine 2000; 25:1782–7.

91. Borchgrevink GE, Kaasa A, McDonagh D, et al. Acute treatment of whiplash neck sprain injuries: a randomized trial of treatment during the first 14 days after a car accident. Spine 1998;23:25–31.

92. Gibson T, Bogduk N, Macpherson J, et al. Crash characteristics of whiplash associated chronic neck pain. J Muscoskel Pain 2000;8:87–95.

93. Jónsson H, Bring G, Rauschning W, et al. Hidden cervical spine injuries in traffic accident victims with skull fractures. J Spinal Disord 1991;4:251–63.

94. Taylor JR, Twomey LT. Acute injuries to cervical joints: an autopsy study of neck sprain. Spine 1993;9:1115–22.

95. Taylor JR, Taylor MM. Cervical spinal injuries: an autopsy study of 109 blunt injuries. J Muscoskel Pain 1996;4:61–79.

96. Bogduk N, Yoganandan N. Biomechanics of the cervical spine part 3: minor injuries. Clin Biomech 2001;16:267–75.

97. Lee C, Woodring JH. Sagittally oriented fractures of the lateral masses of the cervical vertebrae. J Trauma 1991;31:1638–43.

98. Clark CR, Igram CM, El-Khoury GY, et al. Radiographic evaluation of cervical spine injuries. Spine 1988;13:742–7.

99. Woodring JH, Goldstein SJ. Fractures of the articular processes of the cervical spine. AJR Am J Roentgenol 1982;139:341–4.

100. Binet EF, Moro JJ, Marangola JP, et al. Cervical spine tomography in trauma. Spine 1977;2:163–72.

101. Yetkin Z, Osborn AG, Giles DS, et al. Uncovertebral and facet joint dislocations in cervical articular pillar fractures: CT evaluation. AJNR Am J Neuroradiol 1985; 6:633–7.

102. Davis SJ, Teresi LM, Bradley WG, et al. Cervical spine hyperextension injuries: MR findings. Radiology 1991;180:245–51.

103. Ellertsson AB, Sigurjonsson K, Thorsteinsson T. Clinical and radiographic study of 100 cases of whiplash injury. Acta Neurol Scand 1978;5(Suppl 67):269.

104. Pettersson K, Hildingsson C, Toolanen G, et al. MRI and neurology in acute whiplash trauma. Acta Orthop Scand 1994;65:525–8.

105. Fagerlund M, Bjornebrink J, Pettersson K, et al. MRI in acute phase of whiplash injury. Eur Radiol 1995;5:297–301.

106. Borchgrevink GE, Smevik O, Nordby A, et al. MR imaging and radiography of patients with cervical hyperextension-flexion injuries after car accidents. Acta Radiol 1995;36:425–8.

107. Ronnen HR, de Korte PJ, Brink PRG, et al. Acute whiplash injury: is there a role for MR imaging? A prospective study of 100 patients. Radiology 1996;201:93–6.

108. Voyvodic F, Dolinis J, Moore VM, et al. MRI of car occupants with whiplash injury. Neuroradiology 1997;39:25–40.

History, Physical Examination, and Differential Diagnosis of Neck Pain

Eric P. Alexander, MD*

KEYWORDS

• Anatomy • History • Physical examination
• Differential diagnosis • Neck pain

Neck pain is a common and costly problem in Western society. Nearly two-thirds of the US population will experience neck pain at some point in their lives, and at any one time about 5% of the US population has sufficient neck pain to cause disability.[1] Although the likelihood of defining a precise cause of neck pain is low, if the etiology and structural source can be determined, they may be valuable in directing treatment.[2] Patient history serves to identify red flags and yellow flags, whereas the physical examination, guided by the history, serves primarily to confirm those suspicions.

EPIDEMIOLOGY

Spine conditions, including neck pain, were estimated to have a $193.9 billion cost in 2002 to 2004.[3] They are the second most expensive musculoskeletal health care condition, following arthritis and joint pain.[3] In comparison to low back pain, there are fewer epidemiologic studies on neck pain available for review, and risk factors are better established for low back pain than for neck pain.[4,5] Despite this, it is known that many risk factors are common to both low back and neck pain, and that the prevalence of neck pain increases with age and is more common in women than in men.[6,7] In addition, several demonstrated risk factors for neck pain have been identified, as noted in **Box 1**.

HISTORY

When taking a history, the presence of multiple red flags should raise suspicion and indicate the need for further investigation. Although red flags have not been

---

The author has nothing to disclose.
Department of Physical Medicine and Rehabilitation, Kaiser Permanente, Martinez, CA, USA
* 200 Muir Road, Hacienda Building, PM&R Clinic, Martinez, CA 94553.
E-mail address: eric.p.alexander@kp.org

Phys Med Rehabil Clin N Am 22 (2011) 383–393
doi:10.1016/j.pmr.2011.02.005
1047-9651/11/$ – see front matter © 2011 Elsevier Inc. All rights reserved.

Box 1
Demonstrated risk factors and reinforcers for chronic neck pain

- Number of children
- Poor self-assessed health
- Poor psychosocial status
- Past history of chronic low back pain
- Past history of neck injury (even in the remote past)
- Dissatisfaction with work
- Work stress
- Workers' compensation payments

Data from Refs.[8–10]

---

specifically formulated for patients with neck pain, low back pain red flags are commonly applied. Red flags and yellow flags identified by history or physical findings indicate the need for further evaluation with laboratory tests or imaging. These flags are listed in **Boxes 2** and **3**. In any given patient, associated social, psychological, and emotional factors must be considered in addition to, and sometimes more than, organic factors.

When taking a history from patients complaining of neck pain, a few basic qualities of the pain should be elicited, including location, radiation, severity, alleviating factors, aggravating factors, onset, and associated symptoms.

Location: Is the pain in the upper, middle, or lower cervical spine? Is the pain over the spinous processes or over the paravertebral muscles? Is the pain unilateral or bilateral?

Radiation: Does the pain radiate, and if so, where does it radiate? Not only can cervical radiculopathy cause radicular pain but muscle irritation and facet-mediated pain may also cause referred pain in the upper extremities.[11]

Box 2
Red flags for lower back pain (also applicable to neck pain)

- Fever
- Unexplained weight loss
- History of cancer
- History of violent trauma
- History of steroid use
- Osteoporosis
- Aged younger than 20 years or older than 50 years
- Failure to improve with treatment
- History of alcohol or drug abuse
- HIV
- Lower extremity spasticity
- Loss of bowel or bladder function

Data from Haldeman S. Diagnostic tests for the evaluation of back and neck pain. Neurol Clin 1996;14(1):103–17.

Box 3
Yellow flags for lower back pain (also applicable to neck pain)

- Individual factors
    1. Age
    2. Physical fitness
    3. Strength of neck
    4. Smoking
- Psychosocial factors
    1. Stress
    2. Anxiety
    3. Mood/emotions
    4. Pain behavior
- Occupational factors
    1. Manual handling
    2. Bending and twisting
    3. Whole-body vibration
    4. Job dissatisfaction and work relationships

Data from Haldeman S. Diagnostic tests for the evaluation of back and neck pain. Neurol Clin 1996;14(1):103–17.

Severity: Extremely severe pain could be associated with several conditions, including neuralgic amyotrophy, radiculopathy, or cancer.

Alleviating factors: What makes the pain better? A little known clinical sign is the abduction relief sign, in which abduction of the ipsilateral arm over the head may improve the pain in cervical radiculopathy (patients may even say they sleep in that position).[12] Neck pain is typically reduced when patients are recumbent, but if the pain is not reduced by recumbency, then vertebral column infections and metastatic cancer should be considered.[13]

Aggravating factors: What makes the pain worse? Pain that worsens when patients turn and look ipsilateral to the pain can be associated with facet mediated pain or radiculopathy. Pain with contralateral neck motion can be the result of muscle strain or other myofascial pain.

Associated symptoms: Is there also numbness or tingling in an arm or hand? The presence of arm or hand paresthesias along with neck and upper extremity pain may be indicative of cervical radiculopathy, neuropathy, or brachial plexopathy. However, it is common for patients to have mechanical neck pain with coexisting carpal tunnel syndrome. Patients with brachial plexopathy can present with severe shoulder and upper extremity pain, which is then followed by significant weakness and atrophy. These patients do not frequently present with neck pain or worsening of symptoms with head/neck movement. On the basis of history alone, it can be difficult to distinguish brachial plexopathy from cervical radiculopathy.[14]

Onset: When did the pain start? Details about the onset may help determine any sentinel events associated with the pain. Identifying the onset will also help determine the acuteness of the pain and its relationship to trauma (eg, within 24 hours of a motor vehicle accident). Trauma, heavy lifting, repetitive lifting, or long automobile rides may cause radiculopathy.[14]

Nighttime symptoms: Does the pain awaken patients at night and do patients wake up with neck pain in the morning? Any of the possible causes of pain can awaken patients at night, but neck position during sleep must be carefully considered. Do patients use a pillow with good neck support?

Is there pain in the thoracic and lumbar spine? Patients with ankylosing spondylitis may present with nighttime neck and back pain with reduced lateral mobility and an elevated erythrocyte sedimentation rate. Is there stiffness, especially in the morning? Excessive morning stiffness can be present with ankylosing spondylitis as well as rheumatologic conditions, such as polymyalgia rheumatica.

Is there weakness, and if so, where? Potential neurologic causes of weakness include cervical radiculopathy, neurologic amyotrophy, and spinal cord tumor. Weakness in the lower extremities may indicate cervical spondylosis associated with spinal cord compression, tumor, syrinx, or other causes of myelopathy. Is there bladder or bowel dysfunction, which would also be consistent with cervical spinal cord involvement?[14] Is there pain in the lower limbs? Diffuse aching or burning pain may be associated with cervical cord compression.[14] Differentiating peripheral neuropathy, cauda equina syndrome, and cervical myelopathy purely on the basis of the history can be difficult if not impossible.

Previous testing and treatment: Which diagnostic tests have been performed? Which treatments have been completed and were they helpful? This information helps determine which diagnostic tests may still be indicated and provides a basis for a treatment plan. What pain medications are patients taking and are they helping relieve the pain? Have patients been evaluated and treated with a physical therapist?

Past medical history and review of systems: Do patients have a history of coronary heart disease, gastroesophageal reflux disease, or hypertension? If the neck pain radiates to the left arm, is worsened with activity, and improves with rest, then have patients had a cardiac workup? A history of hypertension may preclude the use of some medications such as nonsteroidal antiinflammatories (NSAIDs) or bisphosphonates. Gastrointestinal conditions may also preclude use of NSAIDs. Have patients experienced weight loss or decreased appetite, which could be caused by cancer or a metastatic disease? Are patients taking any lipid-lowering medications, which could cause aching as a complication? If patients are women of childbearing age, then are they pregnant or breastfeeding? This information is crucial in defining testing and treatment limitations. Are patients suffering from depression or anxiety that could be exacerbating symptoms or making treatment difficult? Home or occupational stress is often associated with disability from neck pain.[2]

Social history: Do patients have a history of illicit drug abuse or addiction to prescription medications? Are patients currently working or on disability? Neck pain is commonly encountered in jobs requiring prolonged posturing either at a desk or on an assembly line.[15] Is this a job-related injury? Is legal action pending? If this is a worker's compensation case, then is the case still open? In patients whose accident or injury occurred several months before the initial visit, the consultation may be motivated by legal purposes rather than by desire for diagnosis and treatment. Prospective studies have demonstrated that psychosocial factors are important in patients with whiplash injuries.[15]

Smoking cigarettes is associated with an increased risk of spine pain.[16] It is also important to inquire about patients' social support network, including family and friends.

PHYSICAL EXAMINATION

The basic elements of the physical examination of the neck include inspection, palpation, range of motion, and a neuromuscular examination.

General appearance: Do patients seem to be in pain? Do patients seem calm, in no distress, and yet reporting terrible pain (possible nonorganic origin of the pain)?[14]

Inspection: The muscles of the neck, upper trapezius, and arms should be inspected for atrophy. Is the neck laterally flexed and rotated, as in torticollis? Examine the shoulder for medial or lateral winging or drooping, which may occur with neuralgic amyotrophy, C6 or C7 radiculopathy, or long thoracic neuropathy. Posture is an important factor in causing neck pain. An exaggerated dorsal kyphosis (round back) places the head in front of the center of gravity, increasing the cervical lordosis. The weight of the head in this position is borne by the zygapophyseal (facet) joints and can cause pain.[17]

Range of motion: Range of motion of the cervical spine should be evaluated actively and passively. Is there any loss in range of motion with lateral bending or lateral rotation asymmetric? Is pain associated with neck movement?

Palpation: Examine for tenderness in the cervical paraspinal muscles. Is there tenderness at the base of the skull near the insertion of the cervical spine muscles? Potential causes are tendonitis or occipital neuritis. Palpation and percussion of the neck/cervical spine typically have low yield with regard to identifying a specific process.

Neurologic examination: The traditional neurologic examination for patients with neck pain includes individual muscle group testing of the upper (and at times lower) extremities, a sensory examination concentrating on the dermatomes of the upper extremities, and an assessment of deep tendon reflexes in the upper (and at times lower) extremities.

Manual muscle testing: Manual muscle testing should be performed, at least, in the bilateral upper extremities in the antigravity position using techniques described by the Medical Research Council (MRC) to allow detection of minimal weakness.[18] One commonly accepted scale is the 0 to 5 grading system outlined in the MRC guidelines, with 0 being no movement, 3 representing antigravity strength, and 5 representing normal strength.[14] The examiner should try to determine if the patient is applying full effort; ratcheted, give-way weakness is suggestive of less than full effort. It may be helpful to test the asymptomatic side first to avoid pain and to help the patient understand the motion before testing the painful extremity. In cervical radiculopathy, manual muscle testing is thought by some to be the most important component of the examination to localize the involved nerve root.[19] Upper extremity weakness could be caused by cervical radiculopathy, brachial plexopathy, peripheral nerve entrapment neuropathy (eg, median neuropathy, radial neuropathy, or ulnar neuropathy), poor patient effort, or pain from a tendinopathy (eg, shoulder impingement or lateral epicondylopathy).

Reflexes: As with much of the physical examination, symmetry of muscle reflexes implies normalcy. The biceps reflex may be absent or diminished in a C6 (or C5) radiculopathy, a brachial plexopathy, or a musculocutaneous neuropathy. The triceps may be absent or diminished in a C7 radiculopathy, a brachial plexopathy, or a proximal radial neuropathy. The brachioradialis reflex may be absent or diminished in a C5 or C6 radiculopathy, a brachial plexopathy, or a radial neuropathy. Lower extremity reflexes may be considered, as well as the Hoffman and Babinski reflex. Increased reflexes and the presence of a Hoffman or Babinski reflex suggest myelopathy and the examiner should evaluate further for upper and lower extremity weakness, bowel or bladder incontinence, spasticity, and ataxia.

Sensation to light touch and pin prick: If peripheral neuropathy is suspected, both the upper and lower extremities should be examined. If cervical myelopathy is suspected, the upper extremities and torso should be evaluated for a level of diminished or absent sensation. Decrease or alteration of sensation with sensory testing can suggest radiculopathy, brachial plexopathy, peripheral neuropathy, peripheral nerve entrapment, or myelopathy. When testing sensation in the hand, the cervical dermatomal map reveals that the tip of the thumb is C5 innervated, the thumb and index finger are C6 innervated, the index and long finger are C7 innervated, and the ring finger and little finger are C8 innervated. Each numbered cervical root passes through the foramen above the numbered cervical vertebra (eg, the C6 spinal nerve exits through the foramen between the C5 and C6 vertebrae). As such, a C5-C6 intervertebral lateral disk protrusion may encroach on the C6 spinal nerve emerging through the C5-C6 intervertebral foramen, potentially causing radiating pain from the neck to the thumb.[17] Peripheral nerve sensory innervation in the hand includes median nerve innervation of the palmar aspect of the thumb, index finger, and long finger; ulnar innervation of the lateral half of the ring finger and little finger; and radial nerve innervation of the dorsum of the thumb index finger and long finger.[2]

Several other tests, such as the Spurling maneuver, can be particularly helpful in evaluating patients with neck pain. It involves passively tilting the head toward the side of the painful upper extremity, extending the neck, and then applying a downward compressive force.[20] If this induces radiating pain and paresthesia into the symptomatic extremity (not just in the neck) then cervical radiculopathy is suggested. A positive Spurling maneuver has a high specificity for cervical radiculopathy, but unfortunately, it has a low sensitivity.[14,19]

Shoulder pathology: Patients commonly perceive shoulder impingement as neck pain, so an evaluation of the shoulder can be helpful in determining the pain generator. A basic evaluation of the shoulder includes testing the passive and active range of motion of the shoulder in flexion, extension, abduction, adduction, internal rotation, and external rotation; examining for tenderness in the biceps tendon, rotator cuff tendons, subacromial bursa, and acromioclavicular joint; and testing resisted shoulder abduction. Provocative shoulder tests, such as the empty can test, the drop arm test, the Hawkins-Kennedy test, the O'Brien test, and the apprehension and relocation tests may be helpful in distinguishing shoulder pain, but the diagnostic accuracy of each maneuver to evaluate for a specific shoulder pathology is limited.[21] A more comprehensive discussion of shoulder versus neck pain is covered in another article.

Isolated strength testing of the cervical spine can also be performed. Previous studies have shown decreased cervical flexor strength in subjects with neck pain compared with healthy controls.[22] Cervical flexion strength can be determined in the sagittal, right rotated, and left rotated positions with the chin tucked and subject in the supine position.[22,23] Extensor strength can also be determined with patients in the prone position.[22]

DIFFERENTIAL DIAGNOSIS

Neck pain may originate from various anatomic structures or disease processes. The majority of neck pain is muscular in origin, but usually the precise pain generator cannot be identified. Tendons, ligaments, paracervical muscles, intervertebral discs, cervical nerve roots, and facet joints all have been implicated as a source of neck pain.[2] In addition, neck pain is commonly of a multifactorial etiology.

Neck pain of soft tissue etiology can occur spontaneously, after increased activity, such as a sporting event, housework, a fall, extended motor vehicle travel, a workplace accident, or after a motor vehicle accident. Symptoms are more often unilateral and may be associated with scapular pain. There are usually no paresthesias, although at times patients may complain of unusual sensations. The pain may range from severe to mild. Examination reveals tenderness of the involved muscles, painful neck movements, and painful limited range of neck motion, especially flexion and contralateral rotation with flexion. There should not be any true weakness on manual muscle testing, sensory abnormalities, or reflex changes. Often, diagnostic tests are neither helpful nor necessary unless significant trauma has occurred (eg, major trauma in a young individual or minor trauma in an elderly person).[8]

Degenerative disc disease generally occurs after 30 years of age as a result of the normal aging process, but it can be aggravated and accentuated by trauma.[17] The disc dehydrates and narrows with age, allowing the longitudinal ligaments to be separated from the vertebral bodies.[17] It is difficult to differentiate degenerative disc pain from that of surrounding structures. The intervertebral disc consists of annular fibers, and there is no direct blood supply for the unmyelinated nerve endings in the outer annulus fibrosus. Consequently, damage to the outer annular fibers can conceivably cause pain. With disc herniation, nociceptors in other structures, such as nerve roots, may become activated by compression or inflammation.[17]

Cervical radiculopathy is covered more comprehensively in a later article by Steve H. Yoon devoted to the subject. The location of pain and paresthesias, although helpful in diagnosing a cervical radiculopathy, is not precise in localizing the level of radiculopathy because of the significant overlap and individual variation in nerve root dermatomes.[24] However, common symptoms and associated cervical roots are listed in **Table 1**.

The most common cause of cervical radiculopathy is intervertebral disk herniation and cervical spondylosis, but it may also occur as a result of vertebral column abnormalities, as well as tumor, diabetes, or trauma.[25,26] People in their 40s and 50s are at

Table 1				
Cervical radiculopathy				
Root	**C5**	**C6**	**C7**	**C8**
Pain	Neck, shoulder, interscapular	Neck, shoulder, interscapular, radial forearm	Neck, interscapular, forearm, chest, hand	Neck, medial forearm, ulnar hand
Motor weakness	Shoulder abductors, elbow flexors, external shoulder rotators	Elbow flexors, external shoulder rotators, forearm supinators, forearm pronators, shoulder abductors, wrist extensors, shoulder protractors	Elbow extensors, forearm pronators, finger extensors	Wrist flexors, finger and thumb abductors, adductors, extensors, and flexors
Decrease in sensation	Tip of thumb, lateral shoulder	Thumb and index finger	Thumb, index, middle, ring fingers in some combination	Little and ring fingers
Reflex (diminished or absent)	Deltoid	Biceps, brachioradialis	Triceps	Finger flexor

Data from Honet JC, Ellenberg MR. What you always wanted to know about the history and physical examination of neck pain but were afraid to ask. Phys Med Rehabil Clin N Am 2003;14:473–91.

increased risk for disk herniation, as are those with heavy manual jobs, who operate vibrating equipment, lift heavy objects, frequently travel by automobile, and smoke. There is an antecedent history of trauma in only 14% of cases and a past history of lumbar radiculopathy in 40%.[13] The incidence for the level of disk herniation is

- C6-C7 compressing the C7 root: 45% to 60%
- C5-C6 compressing the C6 root: 20% to 25%
- C8-T1 compressing the C8 root: approximately 10%
- C4-C5 compressing the C5 root: approximately 10%.[13]

Commonly used diagnostic tests for cervical radiculopathy include imaging and electrodiagnostic testing. Asymptomatic patients commonly demonstrate abnormalities on cervical magnetic resonance imaging, and as such any imaging abnormalities must be interpreted in the clinical context.[27] Imaging, as well as electrodiagnosis, are covered in more detail in an article by Plastaras and colleagues elsewhere in this issue.

The prevalence of cervical facet arthrosis increases with age and occurs more commonly in the upper cervical spine, especially at C4-C5.[28] Facet joint disruption may also be at the basis of pain for at least some patients with a whiplash injury.[29] Localized neck pain, neck stiffness, occipital headache, dizziness, malaise, and fatigue are common whiplash symptoms.[13] Localized paracervical tenderness to palpation, reduced range of neck motion, and weakness of the upper extremities secondary to guarding are common findings. Pain from a facet joint can be localized over the affected joint or can radiate into the ipsilateral upper extremity.[30] Facet mediated pain can be aggravated by extension of the spine.[31] Further discussion of the cervical facet joint and whiplash injury can be found in a subsequent article by Alfred C. Gellhorn elsewhere in this issue.

The natural history of cervical myelopathy is variable. Cervical canal stenosis may be clinically silent for a long period of time, sometimes throughout life. Although cervical stenosis and resultant myelopathy can be caused by many pathologic processes, including central disk herniation or trauma and hyperextension in the presence of congenital stenosis (a concern in contact sports), the most common cause is spondylosis.[32] Occasionally disk herniation can lead to acute cervical myelopathy. About 80% of people by 50 years of age and virtually 100% of people by 70 years of age have cervical spondylosis to some degree.[13] The midsagittal diameter of the cervical canal from C4 to C7 is usually about 18 mm. A sagittal diameter of 12 mm or less is generally associated with the development of myelopathy; however, larger dimensions do not necessarily rule out the possibility of developing myelopathy.[13] Cervical spine degenerative changes with resultant osteophytes, bulging disks, facet joint hypertrophy, and a thickened ligamentum flavum, in combination with intermittent flexion-extension-mediated injury, can produce cervical myelopathy in the absence of dramatic cervical canal stenosis. Hyperreflexia and extensor plantar responses (Babinski sign), minimal weakness in the lower extremities, and a subtle gait disturbance are common early signs of cervical myelopathy.[32] Leg discomfort, including burning paresthesia, can occur and may be confused with sciatica. Lhermitte symptom/sign may be observed in some patients. Subtle clumsiness and paresthesia in the hands may be the only initial symptoms and can be confused with median and ulnar mononeuropathies.

Fibromyalgia is a chronic widespread musculoskeletal pain syndrome of unknown etiology, present by definition for at least 3 months. Early in the evolution of fibromyalgia, neck, shoulder, and low back pain may predominate but at its zenith it is usually generalized to such a degree that it is easily distinguishable from a localized spine disorder. In addition to aching pain, symptoms include depression, fatigue, malaise, stiffness, disturbed sleep, headache, paresthesia, and irritable bowel.[33] There is a considerable debate as to whether fibromyalgia is a specific entity or a manifestation of an underlying psychologic disorder, such as stress or depression.[13] Examination of patients with fibromyalgia shows widely distributed tender points to light palpation. Diagnosis, according to criteria established by the American College of Rheumatology, requires 11 such tender points, although fibromyalgia is a diagnosis of exclusion. Further discussion about this topic from a rheumatology perspective is presented in another article by Oberstein and colleagues elsewhere in this issue.

Occult cervical fractures are rare but occur most commonly at C1 and C7. Because 5% to 30% of spinal fractures are multiple and fractures may appear at noncontiguous levels, when injury occurs at one level it is imperative to image the entire cervical spine.[17] Trauma or metastatic disease may result in a fracture or bone lesion. The pain may be severe and neck movement may not be possible secondary to muscle splinting. Polymyalgia rheumatica can cause neck, bilateral shoulder, and bilateral hip pain, and is also covered in detail in another article.

Stingers result from sudden forceful stretch in the nerve roots and brachial plexus as they emerge from the cervical spine. This entity, along with thoracic outlet syndrome, brachial plexus injury, dermatomyositis/polymyositis, and shoulder syndromes are covered in an article by Ozoa and colleagues elsewhere in this issue.

SUMMARY

Careful history and physical examination are essential in the diagnostic evaluation of patients with neck pain. During the history and physical examination, the clinician must be cognizant of signs or symptoms that may indicate a more serious disorder by attending to red flags and yellow flags. The differential diagnosis of neck pain is extensive, and although most neck pain is benign and self-limiting, the real challenge to the clinician is to distinguish serious spinal pathology or nerve-root pain from nonspecific neck pain.

REFERENCES

1. Cote P, Cassidy JD, Carroll L, et al. The Saskatchewan health and back pain survey: the prevalence of neck pain and related disability in Saskatchewan adults. Spine 1998;23(15):1689–98.
2. Honet JC, Ellenberg MR. What you always wanted to know about the history and physical examination of neck pain but were afraid to ask. Phys Med Rehabil Clin N Am 2003;14:473–91.
3. Jacobs JJ, Andersson GB, Bell JE, et al. Health care utilization and economic cost of musculoskeletal diseases. United States Bone and Joint Decade: The Burden of Musculoskeletal Diseases in the United States. Rosemont (IL): American Academy of Orthopaedic Surgeons; 2008. p.195–226. Chapter 9.
4. Cote P, Cassidy JD, Carroll L. The epidemiology of neck pain in Saskatachewan: what we have learned in the past five years? J Can Chiropr Assoc 2003;47:248–90.
5. Harder S, Veilleux M, Suissa S, et al. The effect of socio-demographic and crash-related factors on the prognosis of whiplash. J Clin Epidemiol 1998;51:377–84.
6. Rubin DI. Epidemiology and risk factors for spine pain. Neurol Clin 2007;25:353–71.

7. Cote P, Cassidy JD, Carrole J, et al. The factors associated with neck pain and its related disability in the Saskatchewan population. Spine 2000;25:1109–17.
8. Croft PT, Lewis M, Papageorgiou AC, et al. Risk factors for neck pain: a longitudinal study in the general population. Pain 2001;93:317–25.
9. Kreuger A. Incentive effects of workers compensation insurance. J Public Econ 1990;41:73–99.
10. Sander RA, Meyers JE. The relationship of disability to compensation status in railroad workers. Spine 1986;11:141–3.
11. Travell JG, Simmons DG. Myofascial pain and dysfunction: the trigger point manual. Baltimore (MD): Williams & Wilkins; 1983. p. 23.
12. Fast A, Parikh S, Marin EL. The shoulder abduction relief sign in cervical radiculopathy. Arch Phys Med Rehabil 1989;70(5):402–3.
13. Levin KH, Covington EC, Devereaux MW, et al. Neck and low back pain, vol. 7. New York: Continuum; 2001. p. 1–205.
14. Ellenberg MR, Honet JC. Clinical pearls in cervical radiculopathy. Phys Med Rehabil Clin N Am 1996;7(3):487–508.
15. Drotting M, Staff PH, Levin L, et al. Acute emotional response to common whiplash predicts subsequent pain complaints: a prospective study of 107 subjects sustaining whiplash injury. Nord J Psychiatry 1995;49:293–9.
16. Zvolensky MJ, McMillan K, Gonzalez A, et al. Chronic pain and cigarette smoking and nicotine dependence among a representative sample of audits. Nicotine Tob Res 2009;11(12):1407–14.
17. Cailliet R, Ananthalkrishnan D, Burns S. Neck pain: anatomy pathophysiology, and diagnosis. In: O'Young BJ, Young MA, Stiens SA, editors. Physical medicine and rehabilitation secrets. 3rd edition. Elsevier Health Sciences; 2008. p. 319–22.
18. Medical Research Council (MRC). Aids to the investigation of peripheral nerve injuries. War Memorandum #7, Revised. 2nd edition. London: Her Majesty's Stationary Office; 1943.
19. Viikaari-Juntara E, Porras M, Laasonen EM. Validity of clinical tests in the diagnosis of root compression in cervical disk disease. Spine 1989;14:253–7.
20. Spurling RG. Lesions of cervical intervertebral disk. Springfield: Charles C. Thomas; 1956. p. 47.
21. Hegedus EJ, Good A, Campbell S, et al. Physical examination tests of the shoulder: a systematic review with meta-analysis of individual tests. Br J Sports Med 2008;42(2):80–92.
22. Silverman JL, Rodriquez AA, Agre JC. Quantitative cervical flexor strength in healthy subjects and in subjects with mechanical neck pain. Arch Phys Med Rehabil 1991;72:679–81.
23. Rodriquez AA, Burns SP. Assessment of chronic neck pain and a brief trial of cervical strengthening. Am J Phys Med Rehabil 2008;87(11):903–9.
24. Yoss RE, Corbin KB, McCathy CS, et al. Significant of symptoms and signs in localization of involved root in cervical disk protrusion. Neurology 1957;7:673–83.
25. Hanakita J, Suwa H, Namura S, et al. The significance of the cervical soft disk herniation in the ossification of the posterior longitudinal ligament. Spine 1994;19(4):412–8.
26. Algren B, Garfen S. Cervical radiculopathy. Orthop Clin North Am 1996;27:253–63.
27. Boden SD, McCowin PR, David DO, et al. Abnormal magnetic resonance scans of the cervical spine in asymptomatic subjects. J Bone Joint Surg Am 1990;72:1178–84.

28. Lee MJ, Riew KD. The prevalence cervical facet arthrosis: an osseous study in a cadaveric population. Spine J 2009;9(9):711–4.
29. Lord S, Barnsley L, Wallis BJ, et al. Percutaneous radio-frequency neurotomy for chronic cervical zygapophyseal-joint pain. N Engl J Med 1996;335:1721–6.
30. Winkelstein BA, Nightingale RW, Richardson WJ, et al. The cervical facet capsule and its role in whiplash injury: a biomechanical investigation. Spine 2000;25: 1238–46.
31. Ivancic PC, Pearson AM, Pajabi MM, et al. Injury of the anterior longitudinal ligament during whiplash simulation. Eur Spine J 2004;13:61–8.
32. McCormack B, Weinstein P. Cervical spondylosis: an update. West J Med 1996; 165:43–51.
33. Meleger AL, Krivickas LS. Neck and back pain: musculoskeletal disorders. Neurol Clin 2007;25:419–38.

Evaluation of the Patient with Neck Versus Shoulder Pain

David E. Fish, MD, MPH[a,b,*], Brett A. Gerstman, MD[c],
Victoria Lin, MSIV[d]

KEYWORDS

- Cervical • Radiculopathy • Spondylosis • Rotator cuff
- Shoulder • Arm pain

Neck and shoulder pain are common complaints among the general population, being the second and third most common musculoskeletal complaints, respectively, after back pain in the primary care setting.[1] Although population statistics differ depending on ethnic populations and work-related risk factors, studies have shown that 11% to 14.1% of workers have limited function due to neck pain.[2] In addition, shoulder pain accounts for approximately 16% of all musculoskeletal complaints.[3]

Unfortunately, differentiating between neck and shoulder pain can be challenging, as both share symptoms and physical examination findings. The differential diagnoses of neck and shoulder pain are extensive.[4] For purposes of simplification, the authors adapted an organizational framework for approaching patients presenting with neck or shoulder pain (**Box 1**).[5] This classification includes 5 categories: primary neck pathology, primary shoulder pathology, neurologic disorders, muscle and connective tissue disorders, and non-neuromusculoskeletal disorders. By evaluating patients

The authors have nothing to disclose.

[a] Department of Orthopaedics, Physical Medicine and Rehabiliation, The UCLA Spine Center, David Geffen School of Medicine at UCLA, Los Angeles, CA, USA

[b] Division of Interventional Physiatry, Physical Medicine and Rehabiliation, The UCLA Spine Center, David Geffen School of Medicine at UCLA, Los Angeles, USA

[c] UCLA/WLA VA PM&R Pain Medicine Fellowship Program, Department of Physical Medicine & Rehabilitation (117), David Geffen School of Medicine at UCLA, 11301 Wilshire Boulevard, Los Angeles, CA 90073, USA

[d] David Geffen School of Medicine at UCLA, Office of the Dean-Student Affairs, Box 951720, 12-159 CHS Los Angeles, CA 90095-1720, USA

* Corresponding author. Department of Orthopaedics, The UCLA Spine Center David Geffen School of Medicine at UCLA, Los Angeles, 1245 16th Street Tower Building 7th Floor, Room 715, Santa Monica, CA 90404.

E-mail address: dfish@mednet.ucla.edu

Box 1
Neck/shoulder pain etiology classification

Primary Neck Pathology

- Cervical facet arthropathy
- Cervical discogenic pain syndrome
- Atlantoaxial instability
- Cervical sprain/strain

Primary Shoulder Pathology

- Rotator cuff tendinopathy
- Rotator cuff tear
- Bicipital tendonitis
- Glenohumeral arthritis
- Glenoid labrum tear
- Acromioclavicular (AC) joint arthropathy
- Glenohumeral instability

Neurologic Disorders

- Cervical myelopathy
- Brachial plexopathy
- Brachial neuritis
- Thoracic outlet syndrome
- Cervical radiculopathy
- Peripheral mononeuropathy
  - Suprascapular
  - Long thoracic
  - Spinal accessory
  - Occipital neuralgia

Muscle and Connective Tissue Disorders

- Myofascial pain syndrome
- Fibromyalgia
- Polymyalgia rheumatica

Non-Neuromusculoskeletal Disorders

- Pancoast tumor
- Ischemic chest pain
- Vertebral artery dissection
- Dental pain
- Pneumonia
- Peptic ulcer

within this framework, the authors hope that the vast array of diagnoses that should be considered is easier to diagnose, manage, and treat.

With a detailed and appropriate history, along with a comprehensive physical examination, practitioners should be able to formulate a manageable differential, helping to guide diagnostic testing and treatment options.

PATIENT HISTORY

On initial evaluation, the chief complaint (ie, pain, weakness, instability, limited range of motion [ROM]) should be considered in conjunction with any pain patterns and functional deficits. A visual analog scale (VAS) from 0 to 10 can be used to determine the patient's perceived level of pain. The VAS scale has been shown to be more useful in patients with subacute rather than chronic pain, therefore, caution should be used in the chronic pain population.[6] Anatomic pain drawings can also be helpful in communicating patterns, quality, and locations of pain, and may serve to monitor patients' symptoms as treatment progresses.

General Considerations

The classic cervical pathology related to trauma is "whiplash." It is the most common sequela of nonfatal car injuries and provides significant clinical challenges. The severity of the trauma is often not correlated with the seriousness of the clinical problems, and the exact underlying cause of whiplash's symptomatology is rarely identified.[7] One of the current theories regarding whiplash is facet joint strain leading to a myriad of other secondary symptoms.[8,9] A more detailed discussion of whiplash is discussed elsewhere in this issue. Many other cervical disorders have insidious onset in the absence of trauma.

Defining the exact onset of pain with primary shoulder pathology can be difficult, particularly with overuse injuries. At risk are athletes who endure repetitive overhead motions and individuals who put repetitive strain on the shoulder during activities of daily living (ADL) or work-related tasks. Specifically, rotator cuff injuries are commonly associated with overuse in overhead athletes or workers such as mechanics who put daily strain on their rotator cuff. Labral tears with or without glenohumeral instability may be traumatic or insidious from repetitive microtrauma. Snyder and colleagues[10] reported that a compressive force or traction injury to the affected extremity was the most common mechanism of injury in patients suffering a superior labral tear, anterior to posterior (SLAP lesion); however, 21% of their patients had insidious onset of injury. Moreover, most throwing athletes examined by Andrews and colleagues[11] did not report any distinct traumatic event.

Glenohumeral (GH) instability can occur as a result of trauma or insidiously. GH instability is the result of imbalance between the surrounding muscular and capsular structures of the glenohumeral joint. When associated with trauma, GH instability commonly occurs after a fall on the outstretched hand (FOOSH). This injury forces the arm into abduction and external rotation, levering the humeral head out of the glenoid cavity. Activities associated with this injury include contact sports, falls from heights, and motor vehicle accidents. Atraumatic instability can present as a sense of subluxation or looseness with ADL, and should provoke further inquiry and evaluation for a multidirectional pattern of laxity, particularly if bilateral or posterior.[12] AC joint pathology most commonly involves a fall directly onto the acromium, with the arm adducted against the body. Multiple indirect forces can result in AC joint injury. FOOSH and trauma involving downward force on the upper extremity have also been implicated in AC joint injuries.[13,14]

Primary neuropathic causes of neck and shoulder pain can also present with either acute or insidious onset. Trauma is a common cause of an acute presentation of neuropathic pain.[15–18] Specifically, falls are implicated in cervical myelopathy (fall with exaggerated cervical extension),[17] traumatic brachial neuritis (cervical extension, rotation, lateral bending, and depression or hyperabduction of the shoulder), or cervical radiculopathy due to disc herniation (cervical extension with associated lateral bending, rotation, or axial loading). The rare exception of nontraumatic acute onset of neuropathic pain is brachial neuritis. These patients present with acute onset of severe pain that may follow recent illness, surgery, immunization, or even trauma.[19,20] Up to two-thirds of cases begin at night. In 25% to 50% of patients, history reveals a prior viral illness or vaccination. Some patients may report recent trauma, severe exercise, surgery, infection, or immunization.[21] Overhead athletes such as baseball pitchers, volleyball players, archers, and swimmers can develop insidious traction-related neuropathies including neuropathies of the long thoracic,[15,22] suprascapular,[23,24] and spinal accessory nerves.[25,26]

Myofascial neck pain can occur in the setting of almost any pathology involving the cervical spine or shoulder. There is no classic presentation, as patients may present with a history of acute trauma associated with persistent muscular pain, or without a clear antecedent accident or injury. Patients may also present with symptoms in the setting of poor posture or poor ergonomic set-ups in the workplace.

If patients present with pain after relatively minor trauma that includes some degree of cervical distortion,[27] one must always consider the diagnosis of vertebral artery dissection (VAD) as it can be fatal. Of greatest relevance is those patients presenting after manual spinal manipulation,[28] as this has been proved to be a risk factor for developing VAD.

Location

Pain location and radiation patterns may be helpful in formulating a differential diagnosis. Primary cervical pathology without neurologic involvement will most commonly present with axial neck pain extending into the upper trapezius muscles,[29] without any dermatomal distribution. Patients with facet arthropathy will classically report radiation of pain into the occiput, shoulder, scapula, and proximal upper arm.[30] Similarly, provocative cervical discography has been shown to cause referral of pain into the neck, occiput, face, shoulder, interscapular region, and upper limb.[31]

Pain from acute inflammatory shoulder pathology may be difficult for patients to define, as opposed to subacute or chronic pathology, which may present more often with classic pain patterns. Patients with glenohumeral arthritis or labral tears will usually initially complain of a diffuse pain and note that the pain is actually "deep" within the shoulder.[10] By contrast, patients with rotator cuff pathology often complain of pain in the anterolateral shoulder, radiating laterally along the deltoid and upper arm.[5,32] AC joint arthropathy may present as anterior shoulder pain centralized to the area over the joint itself.[3,13]

Peripheral neurologic processes are commonly associated with clearly defined pain patterns,[33] but this is not always the case. In the first few days to weeks of any acute cervical radiculopathy, pain can be centralized to the medial scapula border or shoulder, and may be initially worked up as shoulder pathology.[5] The radicular symptoms may then progress along the sensory distribution of the nerve root that is involved. With higher cervical root involvement (C4–C5), the patient may only present with shoulder pain, making diagnosis even more challenging. Similarly, patients with acute brachial neuritis (traumatic or atraumatic) may complain of shoulder pain before the onset of distal neurologic symptoms. Patients suffering from neurogenic thoracic outlet syndrome, long thoracic neuropathy, suprascapular neuropathy, and spinal accessory neuropathy may also complain of medial periscapular pain.[15,34]

If pain is diffuse and widespread in the absence of recent trauma, one should consider systemic connective tissue disorders. Patients with fibromyalgia may initially complain of pain at a tender point of a single muscle where their worst pain is localized, but further history reveals that the individual's pain may be more global in its distribution. Similarly, patients with polymyalgia rheumatica may first mention shoulder pain, but further questioning may reveal bilateral hip or neck pain as well. Further discussion of these entities can be found in an article elsewhere in this issue.

Exacerbating and Alleviating Factors

Identification of movements and positions that exacerbate or alleviate pain can be helpful in guiding diagnosis and treatment.

When considering primary cervical pathology, pain exacerbated with cervical extension activities implies facet pathology. Conversely, in patients reporting alleviation of neck pain while lying supine with the neck extended, one should consider a discogenic source. Activities that that increase intradiscal pressure (lifting and Valsalva maneuver) or are associated with vibrational stress (riding in a car or train) have been associated with degenerative disease as well.[35]

Overhead movements or overuse may exacerbate shoulder pathologies and rest may help alleviate symptoms, but further targeted questioning can be helpful in establishing a differential diagnosis. Difficulty falling asleep in a side-lying position is classically associated with rotator cuff tendonitis/impingement or AC joint arthrophy.[3,32] Inquiring about distinct arm positions that exacerbate or alleviate pain may help identify underlying shoulder instability.[3] Patients with instability report improvement with the affected arm supported and exacerbation with the affected arm in a dependent position.[3,36]

Patients with cervical radiculopathy may complain of increased pain with cervical extension, lateral bending, or rotation toward the symptomatic side, all of which are theorized to narrow the foramen.[18,33] Conversely, radicular symptoms may be alleviated by abducting the shoulder and placing the hand behind the head. This maneuver is thought to relieve symptoms by decreasing tension at the nerve root. Neuropathic diagnoses believed to be due to traction neuropathies are difficult to differentiate from primary cervical pathologies, as all are exacerbated by overhead movements. These conditions include neurogenic thoracic outlet syndrome, suprascapular neuropathy, long thoracic neuropathy, and spinal accessory neuropathy.

Neurologic Symptoms

Whenever seeing a patient with musculoskeletal complaints, it is imperative to inquire about signs of neurologic involvement such as sensory loss, paresthesias, or weakness. Proximal neck or shoulder pain with upper limb sensory deficits can be the presenting symptoms in cervical radiculopathy, particularly if symptoms occur in nerve root distributions. Other neurogenic and nonneurologic processes can also be associated with upper extremity sensory symptoms. These conditions include thoracic outlet syndrome that can present with vague shoulder girdle numbness or paresthesias, cervical myelopathy that can present with deficits anywhere in upper or lower extremities, and cervical myofascial pain that may be associated with referred sensory symptoms throughout the upper limbs. Facial numbness and dysesthesias should be taken seriously, as they are common presenting symptoms of VAD.[37,38]

Weakness associated with neck or shoulder pain can be differentiated into proximal (shoulder girdle) or distal (intrinsic hand) weakness. Painless proximal weakness may be a sign of suprascapular, long thoracic, spinal accessory, or traction mononeuropathies. Suprascapular neuropathy may result in decreased shoulder abduction and external rotation strength, long thoracic neuropathy in reduction of overhead strength, and spinal accessory neuropathy in weakened shoulder shrug and abduction. Atraumatic onset of pain in the shoulder followed by progressive proximal weakness is suggestive of brachial neuritis. Weakness due to brachial neuritis manifests within about 2 weeks of pain onset and progresses over 1 or more weeks. Several muscles can be affected, particularly those innervated by the upper trunk of the brachial plexus. The supraspinatus, infraspinatus, serratus anterior, and deltoid muscles are particularly susceptible, but many different combinations of muscle involvement, including a pure distal form, have been reported.[20]

Distal upper extremity weakness in the setting of neck or shoulder pain is often assumed to be secondary to cervical radiculopathy; however, one must always consider additional diagnoses. Patients with cervical myelopathy, lower trunk plexopathy, Pancoast tumor, or thoracic outlet syndrome may also complain of focal hand weakness or loss of dexterity.[39]

Associated Symptoms

If considering a primary cervical pathology, headaches, dizziness, vertigo, or nausea should be considered. Cervicogenic headaches are prevalent in patients with multiple types of primary cervical pathologies, especially facet arthropathy and cervical strain. However, vision changes, vertigo, numbness, nausea, and vomiting are usually only associated with vertebrobasilar artery insufficiency secondary to atlantoaxial instability.[27,37,38,40,41] Failure to diagnose atlantoaxial instability can be fatal for any individual, therefore these symptoms should not be overlooked.

The sensations of shoulder popping, clicking, or catching are classically seen in patients with shoulder instability, whether unidirectional or multidirectional.[36] In these patients, associated labral pathology may be present, including tear extension into the anterior ligament and labrum (Bankart lesion).

When considering possible neurologic involvement involving the cervical spine, one should screen for symptoms of myelopathy. Gait imbalance, lower extremity stiffness or jerkiness, and urinary or fecal urgency or incontinence may indicate a myelopathy and should be further evaluated.

In patients with diffuse musculoskeletal shoulder and neck pain and in whom fibromyalgia is being considered, inquiring about other systemic complaints is important. Fatigue is the second most common complaint in fibromyalgia and patients may report frequent nightly awakening and nonrestorative sleep.[42] Also, sensations of swollen tissues and symptoms of irritable bowel are present in more than 40% of patients with this disorder.[42]

Symptoms of venous obstruction (extremity swelling, venous distention) or arterial obstruction (color changes of the extremity, claudication) may be associated with vascular thoracic outlet syndrome.[34,43] Further details about thoracic outlet syndrome are discussed in another article elsewhere in this issue.

Sports and Work Activity

An athletic and work history may be contributory to the diagnosis and management of neck and shoulder pain. In athletes, competition level, positions, and frequency of play should be considered. Similarly, a patient's profession may entail significant overhead activities thus increasing risk for shoulder overuse, or poor ergonomics and extended time at computers may be associated with cervical myofascial pain. This history is also important in managing patient expectations and recommending alterations or adjustments in sport or work participation.

Prior Diagnostic Testing

Inquiring about prior diagnostic testing will limit duplicate testing and delay eventual treatment. Original images with reports are always preferred over reports alone. Physicians should be comfortable reviewing their own diagnostic images.

Prior Treatments

It is important to review all previous treatments a patient has trialed including physical and occupational therapy, medications trialed, previous injections, chiropractic manipulation, acupuncture, and any surgical interventions.

The quality of physical therapy and compliance with treatments can be variable; therefore, further inquiry regarding length of therapy, modalities, and therapeutic exercises done in therapy sessions, and compliance with home exercise programs should be ascertained. When reviewing prior medications, effectiveness, side effects, and reason for discontinuation should be considered. A similar review should be performed for prior procedures or injections. Actual procedure or operative notes are preferable. However, if unavailable, descriptors of anatomic areas, medications, guidance, and benefits of the intervention are important in managing future treatment.

PHYSICAL EXAMINATION
Inspection

Patients with cervical radiculopathy will commonly tilt their head opposite to their affected side, potentially opening the neuroforamina and relieving pain.[18,33] A forward head position can increase strain on the cervical musculature while also limiting cervical motion.[44] Patients with cervical facetogenic pain develop this posture to offload the posterior elements. This forward head posture is commonly accompanied by rounded shoulders (humeral internal rotation and scapular protraction).[45] This positioning may cause narrowing of the subacromial space and predispose patients to rotator cuff impingement, or contribute to the susceptibility for thoracic outlet syndrome.[34]

Inspection of the shoulder girdle and scapula is best done from behind the patient, and side-to-side comparisons should be made. Diffuse shoulder girdle atrophy may be seen in brachial neuritis,[20] whereas more selective atrophy of girdle muscles may be seen with large rotator cuff tears or suprascapular and spinal accessory nerve palsies. Evaluation of scapular winging should be done with the patient at rest and during active ROM. Exaggerated scapular winging in the presence of long thoracic neuropathy (medial winging) or spinal accessory neuropathy (lateral winging) may be obvious at rest; however, subtle winging may only be seen with active shoulder forward elevation or wall push-ups.

Palpation

Tenderness to the trapezius, levator scapulae, rhomboids, supraspinatus, and infraspinatus is commonly implicated in cervical myofascial pain.[46] However, diffuse tenderness throughout the paracervical musculature should not be considered diagnostic for fibromyalgia, as many cervical pain syndromes can present with similar findings. The diagnosis of fibromyalgia should only be made after a comprehensive history is completed, and the physical examination is consistent with that defined by the American College of Rheumatology.[47]

Systematic approaches to neck and shoulder palpation are crucial to maintain consistency. Palpable step-offs of the clavicle may suggest occult fracture whereas point tenderness over the acromioclavicular joint is more suggestive of arthropathy. Point tenderness subacromially or along the greater humeral tuberosity may indicate rotator cuff impingement or tear. Glenohumeral crepitus suggests glenohumeral pathology. In addition, palpation of cervical, supraclavicular, and axillary nodes may reveal masses or enlarged lymph nodes.

Range of Motion

In the cervical spine, flexion and extension movements are greatest at the C5/6 and C6/7 interspaces,[48] lateral bending at the C3/4 and C4/5 levels,[49] and rotation at the atlantoaxial joint.[50]

Because the complex series of articulations of the shoulder allows a wide ROM, the affected extremity should be compared with the unaffected side as a normal reference. Active ROM should be performed first to establish end range of pain-free ROM prior to the potentially painful passive manipulation of the shoulder by the examiner. Patients with primary rotator cuff pathology may have limitations in both active and passive ROM. Pain may limit passive shoulder internal rotation and active abduction as the rotator cuff tendons become compressed under the anterior acromium arch and coracoacromial arch. Alteration of glenohumeral-scapulothoracic motion can be observed, with glenohumeral motion decreasing and scapulothoracic motion increasing to compensate.[51] Unlike individuals with rotator cuff pathology, those suffering from glenohumeral arthropathy may have restrictions in all planes. If restriction in passive shoulder external rotation is greater than internal rotation, the diagnosis of frozen shoulder should be considered.[52]

Neurologic Examination

A thorough neuromusculoskeletal examination should include, at least, cranial nerve testing, motor and sensory examinations, reflex evaluation in the upper and lower extremities, and gait analysis.

Testing of a patient's cranial nerves should not be overlooked in the evaluation of neck and shoulder pain. Asymmetric strength of the sternocleidomastoid or trapezius may be evidence of a spinal accessory neuropathy. This test is particularly important to consider in overhead athletes or those with recent neck dissection[15] as they are predisposed to spinal accessory neuropathy. Similarly, nystagmus noted during extraocular muscle testing may be evidence of an underlying VAD.[40,41]

Motor examination can include testing of all key (C5–T1) myotomes along with thorough testing of shoulder girdle and rotator cuff muscles. If motor weakness is detected, it is important to consider less common causes. For example, true shoulder girdle weakness may be due to rotator cuff pathology or C5 radiculopathy, but possible underlying suprascapular, spinal accessory, or long thoracic neuropathy should not be overlooked. This is especially true for those with relatively normal cervical spine and shoulder imaging. Similarly, weakness in the intrinsic hand muscles in the setting of neck or shoulder pain is commonly associated with C8-T1 radiculopathy; however, clinicians can also consider the less common diagnoses of thoracic outlet syndrome,[34] Pancoast tumor,[53] or cervical myelopathy.[54,55] Muscle spasticity can be a sign of upper motor neuron involvement and should prompt evaluation for cervical myelopathy.

Similar to motor examination, sensory examination of the upper limb may include testing of key cervical and thoracic dermatomes (C4–T1). Individuals with a clear-cut radiculopathy affecting the dorsal root ganglion should demonstrate sensory changes (sensory loss or hyperesthesia) in a dermatomal distribution. On the other hand, patients with cervical myelopathy, brachial neuritis, or thoracic outlet syndrome may present with more diffuse sensory changes.

Reflex testing can include standard screening of the upper and lower limbs along with an evaluation for upper motor neuron signs with Hoffman reflex, Babinski testing, and testing for the presence of clonus.[45] Reflexes should be tested bilaterally to ensure symmetry. The presence of ataxia with gait evaluation is a potential sign of upper motor neuron involvement.

Special Testing

There is a myriad of provocative maneuvers for disorders of the cervical spine and shoulder. Unfortunately, few alone have adequate specificity and sensitivity to be relied on to make a diagnosis.[45] However, multiple provocative tests used in conjunction for a suspected clinical pathology increase the predictive value of the physical examination.[45] Provocative maneuvers listed in **Table 1** are some used in the authors' practice to screen patients presenting with neck and shoulder pain. Findings on provocative testing should be noted in the context of the other parts of the history and physical examination.

DIAGNOSTIC TESTING
Evaluation of the Cervical Spine

Radiographic studies of the cervical spine are routinely done when evaluating for primary cervical pathology. These views are helpful in evaluating for atlantoaxial instability,[63] degenerative disc disease, and cervical spondylosis. However, evidence suggests that plain film imaging is not a strong diagnostic tool for nonspecific neck pain and has more of a limited, adjunctive role in assessing vertebral and spinal cord injury as compared with computed tomography (CT) or magnetic resonance imaging (MRI).[64,65]

When considering the diagnosis of cervical facet arthropathy, injections of local anesthetic into cervical zygapophyseal (facet) joints may be considered.[64,66–68] Pain reduction after cervical facet joint blocks (medial branch or dorsal ramus) is thought by some as diagnostic of zygapophyseal joint involvement.[66] Supporters of the procedure argue that there is evidence that such joint blocks are reproducible, safe, and accurate in diagnosing cervical facet joint pain',[64,67,68]; however, others question their validity altogether.[69,70] There remains a high false-positive rate in the test (27%–63%).[64]

Diagnosing cervical discogenic pain remains a clinical challenge as well. Unfortunately, imaging studies such as radiography, CT, and MRI cannot reveal whether a degenerated disc is a source of pain.[71] Cervical discography has moderate evidence as an accurate diagnostic tool of cervical discogenic pain, but similar to cervical medial branch blocks, their utility remains questioned.[70] A recent study suggested that discography may cause accelerated generative changes in tested discs.[72] Further detailed discussion regarding interventional procedures for neck pain is covered in another article in this issue.

Evaluation of the Shoulder

Although plain film imaging has limited benefit in evaluating a nontraumatic shoulder, radiography is useful when there is a suspicion of instability or dislocation. Radiography of the shoulder should include anteroposterior views with internal and external

Table 1
Special tests

Examination Name	Description	Reported Validity
Cervical Radiculopathy		
Spurling compression test	Passive lateral flexion, extensions and compression of the head that reproduces ipsilateral radicular symptoms distant from the neck	Sensitivity: 40%–60%[56] Specificity: 92%–100%[56]
Thoracic Outlet Syndrome		
Roos test	Open and closing of fists at moderate speed for 3 min with arms and elbows flexed 90°. Positive test reproduces patient's usual symptoms	Not reported
Adson test	Inspiration, chin elevation, and head rotation to affected side. Positive test is alteration or obliteration of radial pulse	Sensitivity: 94%[57] Specificity: 18%–87%[57]
Supraspinatus Tear		
Empty can test	With the arm at 90° of abduction, neutral rotation, and 30° of internal rotation; resistance testing is performed. Positive test is pain and weakness	Sensitivity:71%[41] Specificity:74%[41]
Subacromial Impingement/Rotator Cuff Tendonitis		
Hawkins test	Forward flexion of the humerus to 90° and forcibly internally rotating the shoulder. Positive test if reproduction of shoulder symptoms	Sensitivity: 88%–92%[58,59] Specificity: 25%–44%[58,59]
Neer test	Elevation of the arm in internal rotation to 180°. Positive test if reproduction of shoulder symptoms	Sensitivity: 75%–89%[58,59] Specificity: 31%–51%[58,59]
Acromioclavicular Arthropathy		
Apley scarf test	Passively adduct the arm across the body with the arm forward flexed at 90°. Positive test if pain centralized to the anterior shoulder	Not reported
Anterior Glenohumeral Instability		
Apprehension test	With the patient in the supine position, the shoulder is passively moved to external rotation in the abducted position. Forward pressure is applied to the posterior aspect of the humeral head. Positive test if patient complains of pain or apprehension in the shoulder	Not reported
Relocation test	After the patient feels pain or apprehension in the shoulder during Apprehension test, the examiner applies posteriorly directed force to the anterior shoulder. Positive test if symptoms of pain or instability are relieved	Not reported
Labral Tear		
O'Brien test	With the patient's arm forward flexed 90°, adducted 10°–15°, internally rotated, and elbow fully extended; the examiner applies downward force. Positive test if pain or painful clicking reported	Sensitivity: 67%–100%[60–62] Specificity: 41%–99%[60–62]

humeral rotation along with an axillary lateral view.[73] MRI is helpful in evaluating bone and soft tissue abnormalities within the shoulder joint.

For diagnosing rotator-cuff pathology, ultrasonography (US), MRI, and magnetic resonance angiography (MRA) are available as effective diagnostic tools. There is evidence that US and MRI have comparable accuracy of 87% sensitivity, and specificity of more than 90% in the evaluation of a full-thickness rotator cuff tear.[74] The advantages of US over MRI are that US is portable, cost effective, and better tolerated by the patient. In addition, US is dynamic and allows for interaction with the patient to optimize diagnostic yield, but the test is highly operator dependant.[73,74] Thus, US is appropriate as a first-line test for rotator cuff tear if the necessary skills are available. For partial-thickness tears, some studies suggest that US and MRA may be more accurate than MRI.[73]

To assess for labral tears, MRA and CT arthrography (CTA) are useful, though CTA is more cost effective.[73,75] MRA, using MRI technology with intra-articular contrast, has the most diagnostic efficacy in assessing labrum, ligament, and rotator cuff tears within the shoulder joint.[11,73] Although MRAs are more expensive than other diagnostic tests commonly used for evaluation of shoulder pain, its cost effectiveness rises as the prevalence of labral tears in a patient population increases.[74]

Evaluation of Neurologic Involvement

When suspecting a neurologic disorder, further diagnostic testing including neuroimaging and electrodiagnostic testing may be warranted. MRI is the most useful diagnostic test in patients with symptoms and signs of cervical myelopathy.[17] CT myelography is the test of choice in patients who have a contraindication to MRI.[76] MRI is preferred over CT myelography because the CT myelogram is more invasive than MRI, and carries increased risk of complications including low-pressure headache, persistent spinal fluid leak, and infection.[17]

When evaluating for brachial plexopathy, MRI of the brachial plexus is considered the best neuroimaging technique available, and is commonly used in conjunction with electrodiagnostics.[77]

MRI testing is widely used as a first-line diagnostic test in the evaluation of cervical radiculopathy.[78] Unfortunately, it has been documented that cervical MRI has a high false-positive rate, with 19% of asymptomatic subjects having neuroimaging abnormalities.[78] Because of the high incidence of asymptomatic abnormalities in spinal MRI, electrodiagnostic examination can determine whether structural abnormalities are of functional significance, or if clinical symptoms and neuroimaging studies are discordant.[18,79] Recent studies have found that needle cervical electromyographic studies can be up to 98% sensitive in identifying cervical radiculopathy if 5 upper limb and 1 paraspinal muscle is sampled during testing.[80] Nerve conduction studies are also useful in ruling out nerve entrapment or peripheral neuropathy that can mimic cervical radiculopathy.[81] Further details regarding electrodiagnosis of cervical radiculopathy are discussed elsewhere in this issue.

If considering the diagnosis of thoracic outlet syndrome, multiple diagnostic tests may be helpful. Radiography can be useful for identifying bony abnormalities (cervical ribs, elongated transverse process of C7), CT/MRI angiograms for arterial compression, MRI for brachial plexus analysis, and US as an adjunctive tool for detection of anatomic vessel abnormalities. Pathophysiology, diagnosis, treatment, and controversies of thoracic outlet syndrome are reviewed in further detail in another article elsewhere in this issue.

SUMMARY

Differentiating among the causes of neck and shoulder pain can be challenging, as the clinical presentations of many of these disorders is similar. Providers are encouraged to develop a systematic, comprehensive, and reproducible approach, including thorough history taking and physical examination along with focused diagnostic testing.

REFERENCES

1. Ferrari R, Russell AS. Regional musculoskeletal conditions: neck pain. Best Pract Res Clin Rheumatol 2003;17(1):57–70.
2. Cote P, van der Velde G, Cassidy JD, et al. The burden and determinants of neck pain in workers: results of the Bone and Joint Decade 2000–2010 Task Force on neck pain and its associated disorders. Spine (Phila Pa 1976) 2008;33(Suppl 4): S60–74.
3. Burbank KM, Stevenson JH, Czarnecki GR, et al. Chronic shoulder pain: part I. Evaluation and diagnosis. Am Fam Physician 2008;77(4):453–60.
4. Pateder DB, Berg JH, Thal R. Neck and shoulder pain: differentiating cervical spine pathology from shoulder pathology. J Surg Orthop Adv 2009;18(4):170–4.
5. Lauder TD. Musculoskeletal disorders that frequently mimic radiculopathy. Phys Med Rehabil Clin N Am 2002;13(3):469–85.
6. Carlsson AM. Assessment of chronic pain. I. Aspects of the reliability and validity of the visual analogue scale. Pain 1983;16(1):87–101.
7. Spitzer WO, Skovron ML, Salmi LR, et al. Scientific monograph of the Quebec Task Force on Whiplash-Associated Disorders: redefining "whiplash" and its management. Spine (Phila Pa 1976) 1995;20(Suppl 8):1S–73S.
8. Siegmund GP, Myers BS, Davis MB, et al. Mechanical evidence of cervical facet capsule injury during whiplash: a cadaveric study using combined shear, compression, and extension loading. Spine (Phila Pa 1976) 2001;26(19): 2095–101.
9. Winkelstein BA, Nightingale RW, Richardson WJ, et al. The cervical facet capsule and its role in whiplash injury: a biomechanical investigation. Spine (Phila Pa 1976) 2000;25(10):1238–46.
10. Snyder SJ, Karzel RP, Del Pizzo W, et al. SLAP lesions of the shoulder. Arthroscopy 1990;6(4):274–9.
11. Andrews JR, Carson WG Jr, McLeod WD. Glenoid labrum tears related to the long head of the biceps. Am J Sports Med 1985;13(5):337–41.
12. Neer CS 2nd, Foster CR. Inferior capsular shift for involuntary inferior and multidirectional instability of the shoulder. A preliminary report. J Bone Joint Surg Am 1980;62(6):897–908.
13. Macdonald PB, Lapointe P. Acromioclavicular and sternoclavicular joint injuries. Orthop Clin North Am 2008;39(4):535–45, viii.
14. Shaffer BS. Painful conditions of the acromioclavicular joint. J Am Acad Orthop Surg 1999;7(3):176–88.
15. Safran MR. Nerve injury about the shoulder in athletes, part 2: long thoracic nerve, spinal accessory nerve, burners/stingers, thoracic outlet syndrome. Am J Sports Med 2004;32(4):1063–76.
16. Olson DE, McBroom SA, Nelson BD, et al. Unilateral cervical nerve injuries: brachial plexopathies. Curr Sports Med Rep 2007;6(1):43–9.
17. Tracy JA, Bartleson JD. Cervical spondylotic myelopathy. Neurologist 2010;16(3): 176–87.

18. Ellenberg MR, Honet JC, Treanor WJ. Cervical radiculopathy. Arch Phys Med Rehabil 1994;75(3):342–52.
19. Suarez GA, Giannini C, Bosch EP, et al. Immune brachial plexus neuropathy: suggestive evidence for an inflammatory-immune pathogenesis. Neurology 1996;46(2):559–61.
20. England JD, Sumner AJ. Neuralgic amyotrophy: an increasingly diverse entity. Muscle Nerve 1987;10(1):60–8.
21. Park P, Lewandrowski KU, Ramnath S, et al. Brachial neuritis: an under-recognized cause of upper extremity paresis after cervical decompression surgery. Spine (Phila Pa 1976) 2007;32(22):E640–4.
22. Schultz JS, Leonard JA Jr. Long thoracic neuropathy from athletic activity. Arch Phys Med Rehabil 1992;73(1):87–90.
23. Ferretti A, De Carli A, Fontana M. Injury of the suprascapular nerve at the spino-glenoid notch. The natural history of infraspinatus atrophy in volleyball players. Am J Sports Med 1998;26(6):759–63.
24. Burkhart SS, Morgan CD, Kibler WB. The disabled throwing shoulder: spectrum of pathology part III: the SICK scapula, scapular dyskinesis, the kinetic chain, and rehabilitation. Arthroscopy 2003;19(6):641–61.
25. Lorei MP, Hershman EB. Peripheral nerve injuries in athletes. Treatment and prevention. Sports Med 1993;16(2):130–47.
26. Foo CL, Swann M. Isolated paralysis of the serratus anterior. A report of 20 cases. J Bone Joint Surg Br 1983;65(5):552–6.
27. Dziewas R, Konrad C, Drager B, et al. Cervical artery dissection—clinical features, risk factors, therapy and outcome in 126 patients. J Neurol 2003; 250(10):1179–84.
28. Haldeman S, Kohlbeck FJ, McGregor M. Stroke, cerebral artery dissection, and cervical spine manipulation therapy. J Neurol 2002;249(8):1098–104.
29. Ahn NU, Ahn UM, Ipsen B, et al. Mechanical neck pain and cervicogenic headache. Neurosurgery 2007;60(1 Supp11):S21–7.
30. Dwyer A, Aprill C, Bogduk N. Cervical zygapophyseal joint pain patterns. I: a study in normal volunteers. Spine (Phila Pa 1976) 1990;15(6):453–7.
31. Slipman CW, Plastaras C, Patel R, et al. Provocative cervical discography symptom mapping. Spine J 2005;5(4):381–8.
32. Blevins FT. Rotator cuff pathology in athletes. Sports Med 1997;24(3):205–20.
33. Abbed KM, Coumans JV. Cervical radiculopathy: pathophysiology, presentation, and clinical evaluation. Neurosurgery 2007;60(1 Supp11):S28–34.
34. Mackinnon SE, Novak CB. Thoracic outlet syndrome. Curr Probl Surg 2002; 39(11):1070–145.
35. Windsor R, Nieves RA, Sullivan KP, et al. Cervical discogenic pain syndrome. 2009. Available at: Emedicine.com. Published April 24, 2009. Accessed November 10, 2010.
36. Illyes A, Kiss RM. Electromyographic analysis in patients with multidirectional shoulder instability during pull, forward punch, elevation and overhead throw. Knee Surg Sports Traumatol Arthrosc 2007;15(5):624–31.
37. Saeed AB, Shuaib A, Al-Sulaiti G, et al. Vertebral artery dissection: warning symptoms, clinical features and prognosis in 26 patients. Can J Neurol Sci 2000;27(4):292–6.
38. Debette S, Leys D. Cervical-artery dissections: predisposing factors, diagnosis, and outcome. Lancet Neurol 2009;8(7):668–78.
39. Huang JH, Zager EL. Thoracic outlet syndrome. Neurosurgery 2004;55(4): 897–902 [discussion: 902–3].

40. Garry D, Forrest-Hay A. A headache not to be sneezed at. Emerg Med J 2009; 26(5):384–5.
41. Kim YK, Schulman S. Cervical artery dissection: pathology, epidemiology and management. Thromb Res 2009;123(6):810–21.
42. Yunus MB. Role of central sensitization in symptoms beyond muscle pain, and the evaluation of a patient with widespread pain. Best Pract Res Clin Rheumatol 2007;21(3):481–97.
43. Hood DB, Kuehne J, Yellin AE, et al. Vascular complications of thoracic outlet syndrome. Am Surg 1997;63(10):913–7.
44. Walmsley RP, Kimber P, Culham E. The effect of initial head position on active cervical axial rotation range of motion in two age populations. Spine (Phila Pa 1976) 1996;21(21):2435–42.
45. Malanga G, Nadler S, editors. Musculoskeletal physical examination: an evidence based approach. Philadelphia: Elsevier Mosby; 2006.
46. Duyur Cakit B, Genc H, Altuntas V, et al. Disability and related factors in patients with chronic cervical myofascial pain. Clin Rheumatol 2009;28(6):647–54.
47. Wolfe F, Smythe HA, Yunus MB, et al. The American College of Rheumatology 1990 criteria for the classification of fibromyalgia. Report of the Multicenter Criteria Committee. Arthritis Rheum 1990;33(2):160–72.
48. Mooney V, Robertson J. The facet syndrome. Clin Orthop Relat Res 1976;(115): 149–56.
49. Sandmark H, Nisell R. Validity of five common manual neck pain provoking tests. Scand J Rehabil Med 1995;27(3):131–6.
50. Aprill C, Bogduk N. The prevalence of cervical zygapophyseal joint pain. A first approximation. Spine (Phila Pa 1976) 1992;17(7):744–7.
51. Poppen NK, Walker PS. Normal and abnormal motion of the shoulder. J Bone Joint Surg Am 1976;58(2):195–201.
52. Sheridan MA, Hannafin JA. Upper extremity: emphasis on frozen shoulder. Orthop Clin North Am 2006;37(4):531–9.
53. Attar S, Krasna MJ, Sonett JR, et al. Superior sulcus (Pancoast) tumor: experience with 105 patients. Ann Thorac Surg 1998;66(1):193–8.
54. Ebara S, Yonenobu K, Fujiwara K, et al. Myelopathy hand characterized by muscle wasting. A different type of myelopathy hand in patients with cervical spondylosis. Spine (Phila Pa 1976) 1988;13(7):785–91.
55. Ono K, Ebara S, Fuji T, et al. Myelopathy hand. New clinical signs of cervical cord damage. J Bone Joint Surg Br 1987;69(2):215–9.
56. Viikari-Juntura E, Porras M, Laasonen EM. Validity of clinical tests in the diagnosis of root compression in cervical disc disease. Spine (Phila Pa 1976) 1989;14(3): 253–7.
57. Marx RG, Bombardier C, Wright JG. What do we know about the reliability and validity of physical examination tests used to examine the upper extremity? J Hand Surg Am 1999;24(1):185–93.
58. MacDonald PB, Clark P, Sutherland K. An analysis of the diagnostic accuracy of the Hawkins and Neer subacromial impingement signs. J Shoulder Elbow Surg 2000;9(4):299–301.
59. Calis M, Akgun K, Birtane M, et al. Diagnostic values of clinical diagnostic tests in subacromial impingement syndrome. Ann Rheum Dis 2000;59(1):44–7.
60. Stetson WB, Templin K. The crank test, the O'Brien test, and routine magnetic resonance imaging scans in the diagnosis of labral tears. Am J Sports Med 2002;30(6):806–9.

61. Burkhart SS, Morgan CD, Kibler WB. Shoulder injuries in overhead athletes. The "dead arm" revisited. Clin Sports Med 2000;19(1):125–58.
62. O'Brien SJ, Pagnani MJ, Fealy S, et al. The active compression test: a new and effective test for diagnosing labral tears and acromioclavicular joint abnormality. Am J Sports Med 1998;26(5):610–3.
63. Kulkarni AG, Goel AH. Vertical atlantoaxial index: a new craniovertebral radiographic index. J Spinal Disord Tech 2008;21(1):4–10.
64. Rubinstein SM, van Tulder M. A best-evidence review of diagnostic procedures for neck and low-back pain. Best Pract Res Clin Rheumatol 2008;22(3):471–82.
65. Goldberg AL, Kershah SM. Advances in imaging of vertebral and spinal cord injury. J Spinal Cord Med 2010;33(2):105–16.
66. Lord SM, Barnsley L, Bogduk N. The utility of comparative local anesthetic blocks versus placebo-controlled blocks for the diagnosis of cervical zygapophysial joint pain. Clin J Pain 1995;11(3):208–13.
67. Sehgal N, Dunbar EE, Shah RV, et al. Systematic review of diagnostic utility of facet (zygapophysial) joint injections in chronic spinal pain: an update. Pain Physician 2007;10(1):213–28.
68. Falco FJ, Erhart S, Wargo BW, et al. Systematic review of diagnostic utility and therapeutic effectiveness of cervical facet joint interventions. Pain Physician 2009;12(2):323–44.
69. Carragee EJ, Haldeman S, Hurwitz E. The pyrite standard: the Midas touch in the diagnosis of axial pain syndromes. Spine J 2007;7(1):27–31.
70. Nordin M, Carragee EJ, Hogg-Johnson S, et al. Assessment of neck pain and its associated disorders: results of the Bone and Joint Decade 2000–2010 Task Force on Neck Pain and its Associated Disorders. Spine (Phila Pa 1976) 2008; 33(Suppl 4):S101–22.
71. Manchikanti L, Dunbar EE, Wargo BW, et al. Systematic review of cervical discography as a diagnostic test for chronic spinal pain. Pain Physician 2009;12(2): 305–21.
72. Carragee EJ, Don AS, Hurwitz EL, et al. 2009 ISSLS prize winner: does discography cause accelerated progression of degeneration changes in the lumbar disc: a ten-year matched cohort study. Spine (Phila Pa 1976) 2009;34(21): 2338–45.
73. Shahabpour M, Kichouh M, Laridon E, et al. The effectiveness of diagnostic imaging methods for the assessment of soft tissue and articular disorders of the shoulder and elbow. Eur J Radiol 2008;65(2):194–200.
74. Naqvi GA, Jadaan M, Harrington P. Accuracy of ultrasonography and magnetic resonance imaging for detection of full thickness rotator cuff tears. Int J Shoulder Surg 2009;3(4):94–7.
75. Oh JH, Kim JY, Choi JA, et al. Effectiveness of multidetector computed tomography arthrography for the diagnosis of shoulder pathology: comparison with magnetic resonance imaging with arthroscopic correlation. J Shoulder Elbow Surg 2010;19(1):14–20.
76. Houser OW, Onofrio BM, Miller GM, et al. Cervical spondylotic stenosis and myelopathy: evaluation with computed tomographic myelography. Mayo Clin Proc 1994;69(6):557–63.
77. Wilbourn AJ. Plexopathies. Neurol Clin 2007;25(1):139–71.
78. Boden SD, McCowin PR, Davis DO, et al. Abnormal magnetic-resonance scans of the cervical spine in asymptomatic subjects. A prospective investigation. J Bone Joint Surg Am 1990;72(8):1178–84.

79. Wilbourn AJ, Aminoff MJ. AAEE minimonograph #32: the electrophysiologic examination in patients with radiculopathies. Muscle Nerve 1988;11(11): 1099–114.
80. Dillingham TR, Lauder TD, Andary M, et al. Identification of cervical radiculopathies: optimizing the electromyographic screen. Am J Phys Med Rehabil 2001; 80(2):84–91.
81. Demondion X, Herbinet P, Van Sint Jan S, et al. Imaging assessment of thoracic outlet syndrome. Radiographics 2006;26(6):1735–50.

Radiologic Evaluation of the Neck: A Review of Radiography, Ultrasonography, Computed Tomography, Magnetic Resonance Imaging, and Other Imaging Modalities for Neck Pain

Scott R. Laker, MD[a,b,*], Leah G. Concannon, MD[b]

KEYWORDS

• Neck pain • Diagnostic imaging • Spine • Radiology

The patient with neck pain may pose a diagnostic dilemma for the treating physician. As with other areas of medicine, imaging is guided by the history and physical examination. The steady advance of 3-dimensional, functional, and nuclear medicine studies make it increasingly important that the ordering physician be aware of the potential benefits and disadvantages of imaging options. This article reviews the current literature on imaging for the patient with neck pain, illustrates several imaging abnormalities, and discusses the workup of commonly seen patient populations.

PLAIN RADIOGRAPHY

Plain radiography of the cervical spine has certain advantages over more advanced imaging techniques. Imaging is inexpensive, quick, and easy to perform, and exposes

The authors have nothing to disclose.

[a] Department of Orthopedics and Sports Medicine, University of Washington, 325 Ninth Avenue, Seattle, WA 98104, USA

[b] Department of Rehabilitation Medicine, University of Washington, Box 359721, Seattle, WA 98104, USA

* Corresponding author. Department of Rehabilitation Medicine, University of Washington, Box 359721, Seattle, WA 98104.

E-mail address: laker@u.washington.edu

Phys Med Rehabil Clin N Am 22 (2011) 411–428

doi:10.1016/j.pmr.2011.03.010

pmr.theclinics.com

the patient to significantly less radiation than computed tomographic (CT) scans. However, radiographs are insensitive to many disorders of the cervical spine, and these disorders may require adjuvant advanced imaging confirmation.

In patients without a history of trauma, plain radiographs are often ordered for the workup of neck pain or radicular upper extremity pain. However, in those with nonspecific neck pain, plain radiographs are unlikely to be helpful in the diagnosis.[1] The history should alert the clinician regarding when further workup and imaging will be necessary. Red flags initially described for acute low back pain can be used in the assessment of patients with neck pain.[1] These red flags include age of onset less than 20 years or greater than 55 years, constitutional symptoms, history of cancer, immunosuppresion, and drug abuse.[2] Evaluation may include laboratory work as well as plain radiographs. Early disease may be missed, and normal results of radiographs should not preclude further workup.

Plain radiographs and advanced imaging may also be obtained for patients with chronic neck pain who have failed a trial of conservative care or for patients with neurologic signs of radiculopathy.[2] The American College of Radiology has developed a set of criteria for the appropriate use of imaging in patients with chronic neck pain.[3] Plain radiographs may not need to be obtained if further imaging with either CT or magnetic resonance imaging (MRI) is pursued. In these cases, a plain radiograph is unlikely to add diagnostic value or alter the management plan.

Routine anteroposterior (AP) and lateral views may show loss of vertebral disk space height, facet arthropathy, spondylolisthesis, malalignment, fracture, and congenital osseous abnormalities. Oblique views are often ordered to evaluate the foramen, but this is highly dependent on patient positioning. The findings are more conclusive with CT and MRI. Flexion-extension views may be added to evaluate for instability, particularly if a spondylolisthesis is found on lateral views. Greater than 3.5 mm of translational displacement or 20° of angular motion is significant and indicates instability.[4] Dynamic views are also obtained if the patient has a history of prior surgical fusion, rheumatoid arthritis (RA), down syndrome (DS), or other known cervical diseases. These views need not be ordered routinely in the absence of any of the above-mentioned conditions. A recent study indicates that in patients with no history of cervical spine abnormality, flexion-extension views do not alter the clinical management of patients, even in the presence of instability, because decisions to operate are based on symptoms rather than imaging results. These views are, however, helpful in surgical planning.[5] The open-mouth odontoid view is needed if there is a history of trauma, or in the presence of disorders that affect the atlantooccipital junction. Indications for more advanced imaging include any concern for infection or malignancy, such as constitutional symptoms, immunocompromise, or history of cancer. Neurologic impairment on examination should prompt more advanced imaging.[2] Examples of the normal cervical radiographs can be found in **Fig. 1**.

RADIOLOGY IN TRAUMA PATIENTS

In the patient with blunt trauma, clearing the cervical spine efficiently and accurately is a priority. The National Emergency X-Radiography Utilization Study (NEXUS) criteria were developed to stratify patients into low- and higher-risk groups. These criteria include the absence of all of the following conditions: midline cervical tenderness, altered level of consciousness or intoxication, abnormal neurologic findings, or painful distracting injuries (**Box 1**). Patients who meet all the NEXUS criteria are classified as low-risk patients and may be cleared on the basis of history and physical examination

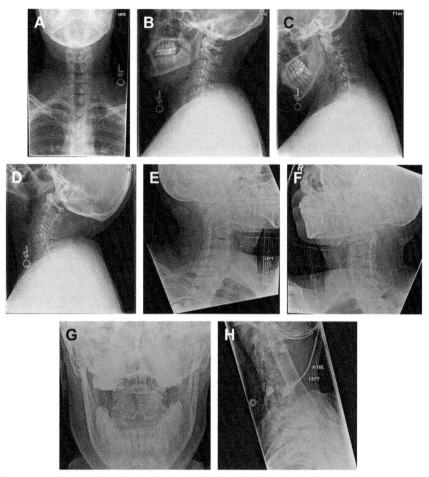

Fig. 1. Normal cervical radiographs. Normal (*A*) AP, (*B*) lateral, (*C*) flexion, (*D*) extension, (*E*) left oblique, (*F*) right oblique, (*G*) odontoid, and (*H*) swimmer's views.

alone. Higher-risk patients require imaging before receiving clearance.[6] Alternatively, the Canadian C-Spine Rules may be followed to determine which among the awake and alert trauma patients require further imaging (**Box 2**).[7] In general AP, lateral, and open-mouth odontoid views are obtained. In the lateral view, the 4 cervical spine contour lines should be evaluated for continuity. These lines include the anterior vertebral body line, the posterior vertebral body line, the spinolaminar line, and the spinous process line (**Fig. 2**). A swimmer's view may be added if the lateral view fails to adequately visualize the C7-T1 junction (see **Fig. 1**), with the goal of preventing the humeral heads from obscuring the spine. With increasing use of cervical spine CT and MRI, the utility of the swimmer's view has been called into question.[8] The open-mouth odontoid view requires an awake and cooperative patient to perform and may not be possible in obtunded or unconscious patients. This view may also be difficult to obtain in the young pediatric population and is not suggested for patients younger than 5 years.[9] Pediatric patients are at an increased risk of higher cervical injuries than adults, and any question of injury to the upper cervical spine in this patient

---

Box 1
The NEXUS low-risk criteria

No midline cervical spine tenderness

No intoxication

Normal level of consciousness

No focal neurologic deficit

No painful distracting injury

Patients who meet all the above-mentioned criteria have a low probability of injury and do not require further imaging.

Data from Hoffman JR, Wolfson AB, Todd K, et al. Selective cervical spine radiography in blunt trauma: methodology of the National Emergency X-Radiography Utilization Study (NEXUS). Ann Emerg Med 1998;32(4):462.

---

population should be evaluated with a CT scan.[10] Flexion and extension views may also be obtained in alert patients to assess for ligamentous injury, although it has been advocated that they are inferior to MRI for this purpose.[11]

Flexion and extension views should be obtained in an active patient in a pain-free range of motion. They should never be taken in the obtunded patient because this increases the risk for progression of injury. A growing body of evidence suggests that CT images should replace all plain radiographs in the setting of blunt trauma because of the low sensitivity of radiographs for identifying clinically significant injury.[12,13] Any patient in whom adequate views cannot be obtained should undergo more advanced imaging. In addition, if any fracture is detected, it should raise concern

---

Box 2
Canadian C-Spine Rules

Step 1: high-risk factors

    Age greater than 65 years

    Dangerous mechanism

    Paresthesias

Step 2: low-risk factors

    Simple rear-end motor vehicle crash

    Able to sit in the emergency department

    Able to ambulate

    Delayed-onset neck pain

    Absence of midline tenderness

Step 3: ability to rotate neck 45° to the right and left.

Patients who meet any criteria in step 1 require radiographs. Patients who do not meet all the criteria in step 2 require radiographs. Patients who are unable to perform step 3 require radiographs.

Data from Stiell IG, Wells GA, Vandemheen KL, et al. The Canadian C-spine rule for radiography in alert and stable trauma patients. JAMA 2001;286(15):1846.

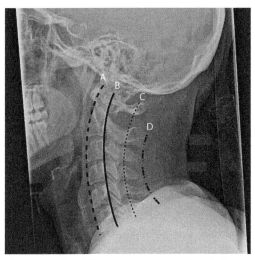

Fig. 2. Anterior vertebral body line (A), posterior vertebral body line (B), spinolaminar line (C), and spinous process line (D).

for concomitant fracture in the thoracic or lumbar spine, and imaging of the entire spine should be performed.

MRI

MRI allows for evaluation of bony detail, marrow signal, malalignment, stenosis, and radiculopathy using 1 test without ionizing radiation. As such, MRI is replacing CT as the first-line advanced imaging for the patient with neck pain. It provides excellent contrast between the spinal cord, intervertebral disks, vertebral bodies, and ligamentous structures and assesses multiple additional aspects of soft tissue or osseous abnormalities.

MRI scanners use radiofrequency (RF) radiation resonant to specific molecules to excite the constituent protons within the tissues. Hydrogen atoms are ideal because they are simply protons spinning across a magnetic axis. The RF pulse causes the protons to align in either one direction or the other based on the magnetic axis created by the scanner's magnetic coil. Whereas the overwhelming majority of these protons cancel each other out, the uncanceled remainder is used to create the images. When the RF pulse is removed, the protons release small amounts of energy as they return to their equilibrium state and spin axis. This release of energy is detected by the coil and is mathematically converted via the Fourier equation into images.[14]

T1 is defined as the relaxation time for the protons to return to this equilibrium net state. T2 is defined as the spin-spin relaxation time, or the relaxation time compared with adjacent protons. Gadolinium is the most common contrast material used in MRI and causes significant prolongation of T1 relaxation times. This material is typically used to assess for infection or tumor or to evaluate postoperative patients. MRI has a reported 92% specificity in detecting tumor and infection.[15] **Table 1** lists the basic differences between tissues as seen on T1- and T2-weighted images. Understanding these differences makes accurate MRI interpretation possible.

As expected, ferromagnetic substances are affected, and all patients should be screened for their presence. CT scans of the orbits or radiographs of the head are

Table 1 Tissue appearances on T1 and T2 sequences		
	Bright	**Dark**
T1	Adipose tissue	Air, edema, infection, tumor, inflammation, blood (acute or chronic), calcifications
T2	Edema, infection, tumor, inflammation, subacute blood (methemoglobin)	Air, calcification, fibrous tissue, hemosiderin, melanin, flow void, protein-rich fluid

Abbreviations: acute, 1–3 days; chronic, >14 days; subacute, spectrum from 3–7 days.

sometimes used to rule out the presence of metallic objects. Pacemakers, hearing aids, and spinal cord stimulators are common contraindications to MRI. Great care must be taken to ensure that aneurysm clips and stent materials are MRI compatible. If confirmation cannot be made, alternative imaging is necessary.

MRI using greater than 1.5-T magnets has been associated with infrequent and temporary sensory, balance, and peripheral nerve disturbance. MRI may be challenging for patients with claustrophobia, in which case anxiolytic premedication or open MRI may be considered. Open MRI scanners are improving greatly, although they still lag behind closed scanners. Surgical devices cause an artifact on imaging, which may make MRI less useful in the workup of instrumented patients.

CT

CT is excellent for complex osseous abnormalities, instrumented patients, and surgical planning (**Fig. 3**). With advancing technology, submillimeter cuts can be obtained rapidly and compiled to create 3-dimensional re-creations. In addition, CT is the imaging modality of choice in obtunded trauma patients when clearing the cervical spine.[16,17]

CT myelography combines the detail of CT scanning with the instillation of intrathecal contrast, allowing accurate measurements of central and foraminal canal diameters. Adverse events associated with myelography are reported to be 4.9% with a cervical approach and 3.4% with a lumbar approach. Patient tolerance is relatively low, and pain after the procedure is common.[18] **Fig. 4** shows images of CT myelography. CT myelography is considered the criterion standard for advanced imaging of the spine, and correlation with surgical findings in radiculopathy is as high as 90%.[19] However, given the radiation involved and the possibility for complications during

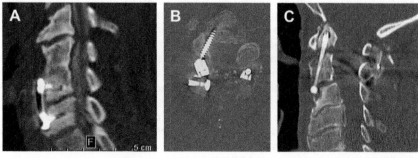

Fig. 3. (*A*) Sagittal CT revealing nonunion of the disk space at C6-C7 junction after surgical fusion. (*B*) Axial CT image of pedicle screw fracture. (*C*) Sagittal CT image of screw eroding into the anterior C3 vertebral body.

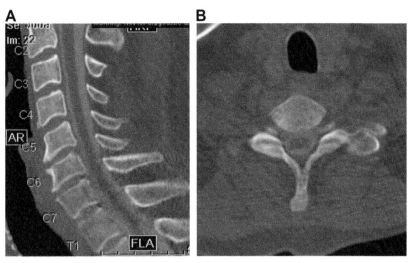

Fig. 4. CT myelography. (*A*) Sagittal views showing C5-C6 and C6-C7 degenerative disk disease. (*B*) Axial images.

the myelogram, MRI should be considered the first-line study if advanced imaging is required in an ambulatory patient with neck pain. CT myelography is now largely used as a supplementary or an alternative imaging modality in cases in which an MRI is contraindicated or extremely accurate bony detail is required for surgical decision making.

DIFFUSION-WEIGHTED MRI

Diffusion-weighted imaging (DWI) and diffusion tensor imaging (DTI) are based on the diffusion properties of water molecules in the cervical spine in vivo. These techniques have been largely used for cerebral conditions including cerebrovascular accident and multiple sclerosis. They are increasingly being used in experimental models to detect early changes in the spinal cord. Technical considerations include limitations based on crossing white matter tracts within the spinal cord, cerebrospinal fluid pulsation artifact, cardiac artifact, and respiration artifact.[20,21] DTI mapping may be more sensitive for intrinsic cord abnormalities caused by cervical spinal stenosis.[22–24] Syringomyelia and presyrinx detection are areas of potential utility for DTI.[25,26] DTI and DWI may offer added insight into the inconsistencies seen between clinical examination findings and MRI findings. **Fig. 5** shows DWI of the cervical spine.

DTI and fiber tracking (FT) are being used in experimental models in patients with spinal cord injury. FT creates a 3-dimensional model based on the use of an algorithm and DTI measurements. FT may reveal more accurate assessment of the individual fiber tracts affected by the injury at levels above the most proximal preserved clinical segment and may reveal partial white matter connections across the spinal cord lesion in patients with sensory-sparing presentations.[27] Early research suggests that DTI parameters correspond to injury severity.[28] DTI and FT have also been used to assess cervical spondylitic myelopathy (CSM) and are more sensitive than MRI in detecting abnormalities corresponding to the area of compression.[29,30] This detection is of significant clinical relevance because it is known that postsurgical outcomes are improved with early recognition of disease.[31] It is unclear at this time if these earlier imaging findings will offer similar clinical improvements. The use of DTI and FT is still

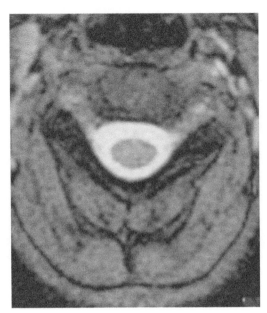

Fig. 5. DWI. Axial cut.

in the experimental phase, although these techniques show promise in adding insight into tract damage that goes beyond the physical examination.

NUCLEAR MEDICINE STUDIES

In the cervical spine, nuclear medicine studies have been used as an adjuvant to image lesions that are suspicious for neoplasm or infection within the osseous structures. Radionuclide studies reflect the function of a tissue because it interacts with the specific isotope. The emitted radiation is acquired by a gamma camera and converted into images by the computer's software. As such, the radiation emanates from within the patient and is detected by the imaging device, and is not transmitted through the patient from an external source.[14]

Single-photon emission CT (SPECT) is the most common type of nuclear medicine study of the spine. The tomographic data obtained rely on 360° imaging performed several hours after the administration of a gamma-emitting radioisotope, typically technetium 99m or technetium methylene diphosphonate, into the bloodstream. These isotopes reflect osteoblast activity and skeletal blood flow. In cases of infection, radioactively tagged white blood cells are the isotope used.

SPECT scan may also have a role in cervical spondylosis and facet pain (**Fig. 6**). Identifying facet pain based on history, physical examination, radiography, and MRI is unreliable. Abnormalities on the SPECT scan in the cervical spine are reported to be 37% in a symptomatic spine pain population, and increase with age.[32] MRI findings of mottled facet synovium, intra-articular fluid, synovial disturbance, and intra-articular facet material have been shown to correlate with abnormalities on SPECT scan.[33] These scans may identify potential responders to intra-articular facet injections in the lumbar spine.[34–36] However, the radiation and the significant cost involved should be kept in mind when using SPECT to guide a relatively inexpensive and safe procedure.[36] To the authors' knowledge, there are no published data on the use of SPECT scans in predicting the response to cervical facet injections.

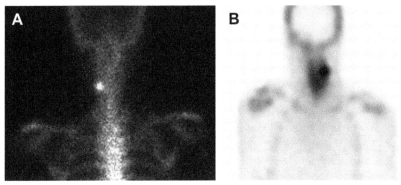

Fig. 6. (*A*) SPECT scan revealing unilateral facet uptake. (*B*) SPECT scan of a cervical metastasis.

ULTRASONOGRAPHY

Ultrasonographic imaging has been gaining popularity in musculoskeletal medicine as a diagnostic tool and for image-guided procedures. Its utility as a diagnostic tool is severely limited in the cervical spine, given its inability to image through bone into the central canal or intervertebral foramen. As an injection-guidance tool, it has been successfully studied for intervertebral facet injections, medial branch blocks, and RF ablation.[37–40] It has been used to perform RF ablation in a cadaveric model with confirmatory pathologic analysis yielding positive results in 30 of 34 medial branch blocks attempted.[40] Similarly, multiple sonographic approaches exist for greater occipital nerve blockade.[39]

Ultrasonography has the advantage of not using ionizing radiation and may reduce cost. Ultrasonographic guidance has also been used to estimate target depth during cervical interlaminar epidural injections in live subjects, although not for real-time guidance.[41] Periradicular injections have been performed successfully in a cadaveric model, although live studies still need to be performed.[38,42] Epidurography is limited with ultrasound given the presence of bone. In addition, ultrasonography is extremely user dependent and requires significant experience to use reliably for cervical injection procedures. Ultrasonography also requires the use of both hands by the operator, making needle manipulation challenging when working in the cervical spine.

The main disadvantage of ultrasonography compared with fluoroscopy is the current inability to reliably assess for cervical radicular arteries, which have been implicated as the cause of multiple catastrophic outcomes with epidural steroid injections. This limitation makes its use unadvisable for cervical transforaminal epidural steroid injections. Doppler ultrasonography (duplex mode) can assess for intravascular uptake, although the resolution necessary to observe radicular artery puncture is unknown at this time. The increased accessibility of high-quality ultrasonographic equipment and increasingly higher–resolution scanners may allow this Doppler ultrasonography to become more clinically applicable. At present, fluoroscopically guided cervical interventions using digital subtraction angiography are the standard of care for cervical epidural injections.

CONDITIONS ASSOCIATED WITH ATLANTOAXIAL INSTABILITY

The atlantooccipital joint is one of the most stable joint in the human body, and dysfunction of the joint can be catastrophic. Instability of the joint is commonly seen in RA, DS, Klippel-Feil syndrome, os odontoideum, Morquio syndrome, and connective tissue disease.

RA

Patients with RA are at an increased risk of atlantoaxial disease. In the cervical spine, as in all joints affected by RA, the inflammatory process begins in the synovium. Destruction extends into cartilage and bone and often causes ligamentous laxity, especially at the transverse and alar ligaments.[43] On lateral flexion-extension views, an anterior atlantoodontoid interval of greater than 3 mm is consistent with subluxation, but this condition does not always require an intervention (**Fig. 7**). Values greater than 9 mm indicate a need for surgical intervention in patients with RA. A more accurate measurement of the space available for the spinal cord is the posterior atlantoodontoid interval. Values less than 14 mm correlate with a higher likelihood of cord compression and neurologic compromise and warrant further investigation with CT or MRI.[44] Neurologic symptoms are not always accompanied by pain, and patients with mild instability may be entirely asymptomatic. For this reason, patients with RA scheduled for intubation and general anesthesia should have AP, open-mouth odontoid, and lateral flexion-extension views to evaluate for atlantoaxial subluxation and instability. For all patients with RA, flexion-extension radiographs should only be obtained after AP, odontoid, and lateral radiographs have been evaluated and there is no evidence of odontoid fracture or subluxation.

Basilar invagination, or vertical movement of the odontoid process into the foramen magnum, can also be seen on lateral or open-mouth odontoid views. Basilar invagination of at least 5 mm with atlantoaxial subluxation significantly increases the risk of permanent neurologic compromise, and surgical stabilization is advised.[44] Sagittal canal diameter of less than 13 mm has also been shown to increase the risk for myelopathy in patients with RA and may require further investigation. MRI imaging can reveal pannus formation at the atlantoaxial joint (**Fig. 8**).

DS

DS is commonly associated with craniocervical instability. This association may be because of intrinsic collagen abnormalities or the presence of os odontoideum.[45]

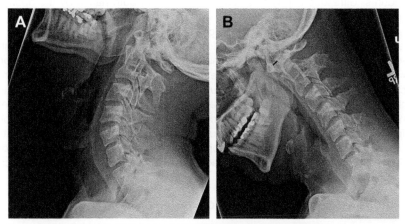

Fig. 7. Increased atlantodens interval (ADI). (*A*) Extension view shows a reduced ADI that expands considerably on flexion. (*B*) Flexion view.

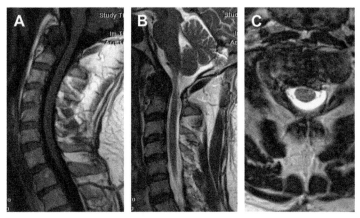

Fig. 8. Pannus formation at C1-C2 region in a patient with RA. (*A*) Sagittal T1 image. (*B*) Sagittal T2 image (*C*) Axial T2 image.

Screening radiographs should be obtained in all children with DS before performing anesthesia or procedures that involve significant cervical manipulation. A patient with DS who is asymptomatic should be screened with AP, lateral, and flexion/extension radiographs. An atlantodens interval (ADI) greater than 4.5 mm is considered abnormal and should warrant MRI evaluation of the spinal cord. Patients with DS p with signs or symptoms suggesting upper cervical neural impingement should be evaluated with screening radiographs and MRI.[46]

The American Academy of Pediatrics and the Special Olympics created a mandatory preparticipation screening for certain high-risk sports. An ADI of greater than 4.5 mm disqualifies the athlete for participation (see **Fig. 7**). This disqualification may be waived with parental or guardian clearance and the written agreement of 2 separate examining physicians.[47,48] Surgery should be considered in symptomatic patients. Although each case is individualized, surgery typically involves posterior instrumentation and fusion.

Klippel-Feil Anomaly

Klippel-Feil anomaly is defined as the congenital fusion of several cervical vertebrae and is often associated with other bony deformities, including scoliosis and Sprengel deformity (**Fig. 9**). Samartzis and colleagues[49] devised a classification scheme dividing patients into 3 types based on plain radiographic findings (**Box 3**). Type I patients have a single congenitally fused segment. Type II patients have multiple noncontiguous congenitally fused segments. Type III patients have multiple contiguous congenitally fused segments. The investigators found that type II and III patients were at a higher risk of developing neurologic symptoms and signs at follow-up.[49] In addition, occipitalization, or fusion of the atlas and the occiput, when combined with C2-C3 fusion causes the greatest degree of atlantoaxial subluxation in the patient with Klippel-Feil anomaly. Most patients are asymptomatic but may carry a higher risk of developing myelopathy, and the decision for surgical intervention is made on an individual basis.[50] Patients with Klippel-Feil anomaly should undergo chest radiography to evaluate for rib fusions and cardiac involvement. They should also have screening renal ultrasonography. If abnormal results are obtained, intravenous pyelography and urology referral should be ordered.

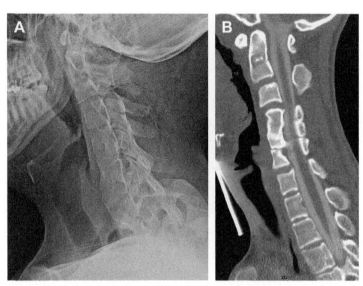

Fig. 9. (*A*) Lateral radiograph of type III Klippel-Feil anomaly consisting of congenital fusion of C4-C7. (*B*) Sagittal C4-C6 Klippel-Feil anomaly.

Os Odontoideum

In os odontoideum, the normal odontoid process is replaced by a well-corticated ossicle that has no continuity with the body of C2 (**Fig. 10**). Debate continues in the literature regarding whether this is a congenital anomaly or the result of trauma at a young age, although it may be that both causes exist in different populations.[51] Os odontoideum is often present in patients with other spinal abnormalities such as Klippel-Feil anomaly and DS. An os odontoideum may be confused with a dens fracture on initial radiographs. The os odontoideum should appear well corticated, with a wide gap separating it from an inferior hypoplastic odontoid process on plain radiographs. This appearance is in contrast to that of a fracture fragment, which demonstrates irregular cortication, a smaller gap, and a normally developed dens. Once os odontoideum has been identified in a patient with AP, lateral, and open-mouth views, the presence of atlantoaxial instability must be assessed by flexion and extension views.[52] The ossicle and the ring of C1 often move as a unit on these views. Patients with neurologic symptoms, or equivocal radiographs or those considering surgical intervention should undergo more advanced imaging.

Box 3
Klippel-Feil anomaly

Type I: single congenitally fused segment

Type II: multiple noncontiguous congenitally fused segments

Type III: multiple contiguous congenitally fused segments

Data from Samartzis DD, Herman J, Lubicky JP, et al. Classification of congenitally fused cervical patterns in Klippel-Feil patients: epidemiology and role in the development of cervical spine-related symptoms. Spine (Phila Pa 1976) 2006;31(21):E799.

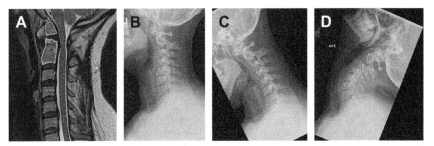

Fig. 10. (A) Sagittal T2 MRI, (B) lateral view, (C) flexion view, and (D) extension view of os odontoideum. Note the subtle motion seen in flexion and extension radiographs.

SPECIFIC CONDITIONS

Several disease states have direct effects on the structure and function of the cervical spine and warrant special consideration. In addition, imaging often reveals unexpected abnormalities that require further workup. The following sections discuss some of these common diseases and findings.

Ankylosing Spondylitis

Patients with ankylosing spinal disorders, such as ankylosing spondylitis and diffuse idiopathic skeletal hyperostosis, have an increased risk of spinal fractures (**Fig. 11**). Most fractures are present in the cervical spine and result from low-energy traumas, such as a fall. Many of these fractures are associated with neurologic injury, although there may be a delay in the development of symptoms.[53] Early advanced imaging with CT or MRI is advocated in these patients.[54]

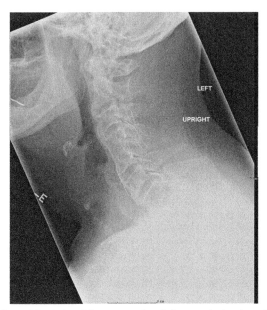

Fig. 11. Diffuse idiopathic skeletal hyperostosis of the cervical spine. Note the bridging osteophytes throughout the anterior cervical spine. Incidental Klippel-Feil anomaly at C4-C5 region.

CSM

CSM occurs when the spinal cord is injured by the aging process of the spine. CSM is the most common cause of myelopathy in adults. MRI is the study of choice because it offers the ability to measure the central and foraminal dimensions and allows assessment of the spinal cord itself. Hyperintensity on T2-weighted images is commonly seen in CSM but has not been shown to be a prognostic factor. Studies have found conflicting results using cord signal as a prognostic factor for postsurgical improvement.[55–57] Hypointensity on T1-weighted image is much less common and is associated with poorer surgical outcomes. Asymptomatic CSM on MRI is not an indication for surgery, although it may warrant specialty consultation.

Chiari Malformation

The Chiari malformation is defined as the presence of the cerebellar tonsils below the level of the foramen magnum. It is often associated with syringomyelia, although the mechanism is not well understood (**Fig. 12**). The resultant symptoms are likely due to pressure placed on the cerebellar tonsils and pressure disturbance on the cerebrospinal fluid. Type I Chiari malformations, the most common variant, are congenital. Patients are largely asymptomatic in childhood but may present with cerebellar signs or headache that worsens with Valsalva maneuver. The associated syrinx may present as a central cord syndrome. Type I Chiari malformations and cerebellar ectopia are seen occasionally on cervical or brain MRI. Symptomatic patients or patients with syringomyelia should undergo surgical decompression of the malformation. The syrinx typically resolves postoperatively and does not require shunting. Malformations that do not correspond to the patients' symptoms do not require surgery, but patients should be educated about concerning symptoms. Cine MRI has been used to help differentiate symptomatic type I Chiari malformations from asymptomatic cerebellar ectopia and to help predict surgical outcomes.[58,59] Asymptomatic patients may be monitored serially.

Type II or Arnold-Chiari malformations are less common and present with more prominent imaging findings and more severe symptoms. They are almost always associated with lumbar myelomeningocele and can present with paralysis, cerebellar signs, and cranial nerve dysfunction. Because of the severe symptoms, these patients typically present during infancy or early childhood. Type II malformations are closely

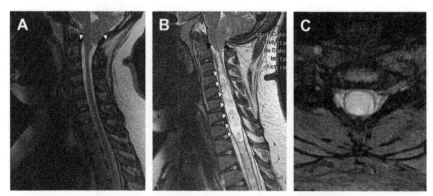

Fig. 12. (*A*) Sagittal T2 MRI revealing ectopic cerebellar tonsils (*white arrowheads*). (*B*) Sagittal T2 MRI of a more prominent type I Chiari malformation (*black arrowheads*) with significant syringomyelia (*white arrowheads*). (*C*) Axial T2 image of the same patient. Note the near obliteration of the central spinal cord by the syrinx.

associated with hydrocephalus and require shunting. Surgical decompression is considered if cerebellar signs are present despite adequate shunt function.

SUMMARY

Imaging the patient with neck pain requires an in-depth understanding of anatomy, abnormality, and the modality being used to perform the investigation. Information gathered from the history and physical examination directly affects the study ordered by the physician. As imaging progresses, isolated radiographs continue to move toward multimodality evaluation of patients with neck pain. Effective use of the full gamut of imaging modalities allows the physician to reliably diagnose and treat the patient with neck pain. Future trends suggest the use of functional imaging to help guide both surgical and nonsurgical treatments.

REFERENCES

1. Rubinstein SM, van Tulder M. A best-evidence review of diagnostic procedures for neck and low-back pain. Best Pract Res Clin Rheumatol 2008;22(3):471–82.
2. van Tulder M, Becker A, Bekkering T, et al. Chapter 3. European guidelines for the management of acute nonspecific low back pain in primary care. Eur Spine J 2006;15(Suppl 2):S169–91.
3. Daffner RH, Dalinka MK, Alazraki N, et al. Chronic neck pain. American College of Radiology. ACR appropriateness criteria. Radiology 2000;215(Suppl):345–56.
4. White AA 3rd, Johnson RM, Panjabi MM, et al. Biomechanical analysis of clinical stability in the cervical spine. Clin Orthop Relat Res 1975;109:85–96.
5. White AP, Biswas D, Smart LR, et al. Utility of flexion-extension radiographs in evaluating the degenerative cervical spine. Spine (Phila Pa 1976) 2007;32(9): 975–9.
6. Hoffman JR, Wolfson AB, Todd K, et al. Selective cervical spine radiography in blunt trauma: methodology of the National Emergency X-Radiography Utilization Study (NEXUS). Ann Emerg Med 1998;32(4):461–9.
7. Stiell IG, Wells GA, Vandemheen KL, et al. The Canadian C-spine rule for radiography in alert and stable trauma patients. JAMA 2001;286(15):1841–8.
8. Rethnam U, Yesupalan RS, Bastawrous SS. The swimmer's view: does it really show what it is supposed to show? A retrospective study. BMC Med Imaging 2008;8:2.
9. Swischuk LE, John SD, Hendrick EP. Is the open-mouth odontoid view necessary in children under 5 years? Pediatr Radiol 2000;30(3):186–9.
10. Buhs C, Cullen M, Klein M, et al. The pediatric trauma C-spine: is the 'odontoid' view necessary? J Pediatr Surg 2000;35(6):994–7.
11. Duane TM, Cross J, Scarcella N, et al. Flexion-extension cervical spine plain films compared with MRI in the diagnosis of ligamentous injury. Am Surg 2010;76(6): 595–8.
12. Gale SC, Gracias VH, Reilly PM, et al. The inefficiency of plain radiography to evaluate the cervical spine after blunt trauma. J Trauma 2005;59(5):1121–5.
13. Bailitz J, Starr F, Beecroft M, et al. CT should replace three-view radiographs as the initial screening test in patients at high, moderate, and low risk for blunt cervical spine injury: a prospective comparison. J Trauma 2009;66(6):1605–9.
14. Adam A, Dixon AK, Grainger RG, et al. Grainger and Allison's diagnostic radiology. In: Adam A, Dixon AK, Grainger RG, et al, editors. 5th edition. Edinburgh (UK): Churchill Livingstone; 2008.

15. Modic MT, Masaryk TJ, Mulopulos GP, et al. Cervical radiculopathy: prospective evaluation with surface coil MR imaging, CT with metrizamide, and metrizamide myelography. Radiology 1986;161(3):753–9.
16. Brohi K, Healy M, Fotheringham T, et al. Helical computed tomographic scanning for the evaluation of the cervical spine in the unconscious, intubated trauma patient. J Trauma 2005;58(5):897–901.
17. Griffen MM, Frykberg ER, Kerwin AJ, et al. Radiographic clearance of blunt cervical spine injury: plain radiograph or computed tomography scan? J Trauma 2003;55(2):222–6 [discussion: 226–7].
18. Chin KR, Eiszner JR, Huang JL, et al. Myelographic evaluation of cervical spondylosis: patient tolerance and complications. J Spinal Disord Tech 2008;21(5): 334–7.
19. Modic MT, Masaryk TJ, Ross JS, et al. Cervical radiculopathy: value of oblique MR imaging. Radiology 1987;163(1):227–31.
20. Clark CA, Werring DJ. Diffusion tensor imaging in spinal cord: methods and applications-a review. NMR Biomed 2002;15(7/8):578–86.
21. Cercignani M, Horsfield MA, Agosta F, et al. Sensitivity-encoded diffusion tensor MR imaging of the cervical cord. AJNR Am J Neuroradiol 2003;24(6):1254–6.
22. Song T, Chen WJ, Yang B, et al. Diffusion tensor imaging in the cervical spinal cord. Eur Spine J 2011;20(3):422–8.
23. Ries M, Jones RA, Dousset V, et al. Diffusion tensor MRI of the spinal cord. Magn Reson Med 2000;44(6):884–92.
24. Mamata H, Jolesz FA, Maier SE. Characterization of central nervous system structures by magnetic resonance diffusion anisotropy. Neurochem Int 2004;45(4): 553–60.
25. Roser F, Ebner F, Maier G, et al. Fractional anisotropy levels derived from diffusion tensor imaging in cervical syringomyelia. Neurosurgery 2010;67(4):901–5 [discussion: 905].
26. Fischbein NJ, Dillon WP, Cobbs C, et al. The "presyrinx" state: a reversible myelopathic condition that may precede syringomyelia. AJNR Am J Neuroradiol 1999; 20(1):7–20.
27. Chang Y, Jung TD, Yoo DS, et al. Diffusion tensor imaging and fiber tractography of patients with cervical spinal cord injury. J Neurotrauma 2010;27(11):2033–40.
28. Shanmuganathan K, Gullapalli RP, Zhuo J, et al. Diffusion tensor MR imaging in cervical spine trauma. AJNR Am J Neuroradiol 2008;29(4):655–9.
29. Xiangshui M, Xiangjun C, Xiaoming Z, et al. 3 T magnetic resonance diffusion tensor imaging and fibre tracking in cervical myelopathy. Clin Radiol 2010; 65(6):465–73.
30. Demir A, Ries M, Moonen CT, et al. Diffusion-weighted MR imaging with apparent diffusion coefficient and apparent diffusion tensor maps in cervical spondylotic myelopathy. Radiology 2003;229(1):37–43.
31. Sampath P, Bendebba M, Davis JD, et al. Outcome of patients treated for cervical myelopathy. A prospective, multicenter study with independent clinical review. Spine (Phila Pa 1976) 2000;25(6):670–6.
32. Makki D, Khazim R, Zaidan AA, et al. Single photon emission computerized tomography (SPECT) scan-positive facet joints and other spinal structures in a hospital-wide population with spinal pain. Spine J 2010;10(1):58–62.
33. Kim KY, Wang MY. Magnetic resonance image-based morphological predictors of single photon emission computed tomography-positive facet arthropathy in patients with axial back pain. Neurosurgery 2006;59(1):147–56 [discussion: 147–56].

34. Dolan AL, Ryan PJ, Arden NK, et al. The value of SPECT scans in identifying back pain likely to benefit from facet joint injection. Br J Rheumatol 1996;35(12):1269–73.
35. Ackerman WE 3rd, Ahmad M. Pain relief with intraarticular or medial branch nerve blocks in patients with positive lumbar facet joint SPECT imaging: a 12-week outcome study. South Med J 2008;101(9):931–4.
36. Pneumaticos SG, Chatziioannou SN, Hipp JA, et al. Low back pain: prediction of short-term outcome of facet joint injection with bone scintigraphy. Radiology 2006;238(2):693–8.
37. Eichenberger U, Greher M, Kapral S, et al. Sonographic visualization and ultrasound-guided block of the third occipital nerve: prospective for a new method to diagnose C2-C3 zygapophysial joint pain. Anesthesiology 2006; 104(2):303–8.
38. Galiano K, Obwegeser AA, Bale R, et al. Ultrasound-guided and CT-navigation-assisted periradicular and facet joint injections in the lumbar and cervical spine: a new teaching tool to recognize the sonoanatomic pattern. Reg Anesth Pain Med 2007;32(3):254–7.
39. Greher M, Moriggl B, Curatolo M, et al. Sonographic visualization and ultrasound-guided blockade of the greater occipital nerve: a comparison of two selective techniques confirmed by anatomical dissection. Br J Anaesth 2010;104(5): 637–42.
40. Lee SH, Kang CH, Derby R, et al. Ultrasound-guided radiofrequency neurotomy in cervical spine: sonoanatomic study of a new technique in cadavers. Clin Radiol 2008;63(11):1205–12.
41. Kim SH, Lee KH, Yoon KB, et al. Sonographic estimation of needle depth for cervical epidural blocks. Anesth Analg 2008;106(5):1542–7.
42. Galiano K, Obwegeser AA, Bodner G, et al. Ultrasound-guided periradicular injections in the middle to lower cervical spine: an imaging study of a new approach. Reg Anesth Pain Med 2005;30(4):391–6.
43. Klippel JH. Primer on the rheumatic diseases. 13th edition. New York: Springer; 2008.
44. Boden SD, Dodge LD, Bohlman HH, et al. Rheumatoid arthritis of the cervical spine. A long-term analysis with predictors of paralysis and recovery. J Bone Joint Surg Am 1993;75(9):1282–97.
45. Brockmeyer D. Down syndrome and craniovertebral instability. Topic review and treatment recommendations. Pediatr Neurosurg 1999;31(2):71–7.
46. White KS, Ball WS, Prenger EC, et al. Evaluation of the craniocervical junction in Down syndrome: correlation of measurements obtained with radiography and MR imaging. Radiology 1993;186(2):377–82.
47. Specialolympics.org. Participation by individuals with Down syndrome who have atlantoaxial instability. Available at: http://info.specialolympics.org/Special+Olympics+Public+Website/English/Coach/Coaching_Guides/Basics+of+Special+Olympics/Down+Syndrome+and+Restrictions+Based+on+Atlantoaxial+Instability.htm. Accessed October 11, 2010.
48. American Academy of Pediatrics. Committee on Sports Medicine. Atlantoaxial instability in Down Syndrome. Pediatrics 1984;74(1):152–4.
49. Samartzis DD, Herman J, Lubicky JP, et al. Classification of congenitally fused cervical patterns in Klippel-Feil patients: epidemiology and role in the development of cervical spine-related symptoms. Spine (Phila Pa 1976) 2006;31(21):E798–804.
50. Shen FH, Samartzis D, Herman J, et al. Radiographic assessment of segmental motion at the atlantoaxial junction in the Klippel-Feil patient. Spine (Phila Pa 1976) 2006;31(2):171–7.

51. Sankar WN, Wills BP, Dormans JP, et al. Os odontoideum revisited: the case for a multifactorial etiology. Spine (Phila Pa 1976) 2006;31(9):979–84.
52. Smoker WR, Khanna G. Imaging the craniocervical junction. Childs Nerv Syst 2008;24(10):1123–45.
53. Hendrix RW, Melany M, Miller F, et al. Fracture of the spine in patients with ankylosis due to diffuse skeletal hyperostosis: clinical and imaging findings. AJR Am J Roentgenol 1994;162(4):899–904.
54. Caron T, Bransford R, Nguyen Q, et al. Spine fractures in patients with ankylosing spinal disorders. Spine (Phila Pa 1976) 2010;35(11):E458–64.
55. Okada Y, Ikata T, Yamada H, et al. Magnetic resonance imaging study on the results of surgery for cervical compression myelopathy. Spine (Phila Pa 1976) 1993;18(14):2024–9.
56. Mehalic TF, Pezzuti RT, Applebaum BI. Magnetic resonance imaging and cervical spondylotic myelopathy. Neurosurgery 1990;26(2):217–26 [discussion: 226–7].
57. Yukawa Y, Kato F, Yoshihara H, et al. MR T2 image classification in cervical compression myelopathy: predictor of surgical outcomes. Spine (Phila Pa 1976) 2007;32(15):1675–8 [discussion: 1679].
58. McGirt MJ, Nimjee SM, Fuchs HE, et al. Relationship of cine phase-contrast magnetic resonance imaging with outcome after decompression for Chiari I malformations. Neurosurgery 2006;59(1):140–6 [discussion: 140–6].
59. Hofkes SK, Iskandar BJ, Turski PA, et al. Differentiation between symptomatic Chiari I malformation and asymptomatic tonsilar ectopia by using cerebrospinal fluid flow imaging: initial estimate of imaging accuracy. Radiology 2007;245(2):532–40.

The Electrodiagnostic Evaluation of Neck Pain

Christopher T. Plastaras, MD*, Anand B. Joshi, MD, MHA

KEYWORDS

- Electromyography • Radiculopathy • Electrodiagnosis
- Spinal stenosis

Radiculopathy is a functional diagnosis implying dysfunction of the spinal nerve root. Although commonly caused by structural lesions, such as degenerative spondylosis, it can also be caused by inflammatory, infectious, or malignant disorders. Structural causes of radiculopathy may be readily apparent through imaging modalities, such as magnetic resonance imaging (MRI) or computed axial tomography. However, MRI is known to be clinically nonspecific, and may not pinpoint the structural cause of radiculopathy. Additionally, infectious or malignant causes may not be readily apparent on standard imaging without contrast. In such equivocal cases, imaging may be complemented by electrodiagnostic testing. Electrodiagnostic testing is a functional evaluation of the nervous system, and allows objective documentation of the chronicity and severity of nervous system disease.

DEFINITION

The needle electrode examination (NEE) is a crucial component of electrodiagnostic testing. It indicates radiculopathy when abnormalities are found in muscles innervated by the same nerve root but by different peripheral nerves, provided that muscles innervated by adjacent nerve roots are normal. Motor and sensory nerve conduction studies are not diagnostic of radiculopathy alone, but are necessary to rule out possible concurrent conditions, such as polyneuropathy or mononeuropathy.

HISTORY AND EXAMINATION

As with much diagnostic testing, electrodiagnosis is an extension of the history and physical examination. However, it can be painful, expensive, and somewhat insensitive. As such, several studies have evaluated the role of the history and physical examination in predicting cervical radiculopathies found with electrodiagnostic testing.[1] Patients with symptoms of numbness, tingling, and subjective weakness were more

See attached conflict disclosures. The authors have no financial disclosures.
Department of Physical Medicine & Rehabilitation, Penn Spine Center, University of Pennsylvania, 3400 Spruce Street, Ground Floor, White Building, Philadelphia, PA 19104, USA
* Corresponding author.
E-mail address: christopher.plastaras@uphs.upenn.edu

Phys Med Rehabil Clin N Am 22 (2011) 429–438
doi:10.1016/j.pmr.2011.02.012
1047-9651/11/$ – see front matter © 2011 Elsevier Inc. All rights reserved.

than twice as likely to have abnormal electromyogram (EMG) findings. However, none of these symptoms significantly or specifically predicted an electrodiagnostic test result diagnostic of radiculopathy. In contrast, the presence of weakness, abnormal reflexes, or abnormal sensation on physical examination is associated with greater than four times likelihood of having an abnormal electrodiagnostic study, and greater than two times likelihood of confirming a cervical radiculopathy. A particularly valuable physical examination finding is an abnormal biceps reflex, which increases to 10 the odds ratio of making an EMG diagnosis of cervical radiculopathy. In general, the combination of having weakness and a reduced reflex is a strong predictor of both an abnormal electrodiagnostic study and of electrodiagnostic radiculopathy, specifically. Notably, up to 48% of individuals have a normal physical examination with abnormal electrodiagnostic results, emphasizing the physical examination's lack of sensitivity when using electrodiagnosis as a gold standard, and the value of electrodiagnostic studies in individuals with normal physical examinations.[1]

NERVE ROOT VARIATION

The electrodiagnosis of radiculopathy relies on a myotomal pattern of abnormalities found on NEE. However, variation in the anatomic pattern of nerve roots is known to exist and must be accounted for in the interpretation of the NEE. In a study of 200 fetuses, 107 (53.5%) showed significant variation in the arrangement of the brachial plexus.[2] The most common variants of brachial plexus organization are described as "prefixed" (up to 48%) and "postfixed" (0.5%–4%).[2,3] These have been variously defined[4] and emphasize the contributions of the C4 and T2 roots. A prefixed plexus is characterized by a C4 branch that is larger than the branch from T2.[5] As such, C4 may contribute to the innervation of the shoulder girdle musculature, which is more typically C5. In contrast, a postfixed plexus contains a large contribution from T2, and a relatively small contribution from C4.[5] Such normal variations in peripheral nervous system anatomy must be accounted for in the performance of the NEE.

SENSITIVITY OF EMG

The sensitivity of EMG in detecting radiculopathy is limited by several factors. Because the procedure is targeted exclusively toward motor axons, radiculopathies with predominant sensory root involvement do not elicit any needle electrode abnormalities.[6] Demyelinating disease may be detected on the NEE by changes in motor unit recruitment; however, significant demyelination at the level of the nerve root is uncommon.[6] The electrodiagnostic confirmation of radiculopathy requires abnormal findings in a myotomal pattern. Such identification may not occur if axonal compromise is not severe or widespread enough to be detected by the needle electrode. Additionally, the appearance of fibrillation potentials is very time dependent. If NEE is done too early, fibrillations may not yet have developed. If done too late (ie, >6 months after the onset of cervical radiculopathies),[7] fibrillations may disappear. Finally, even if denervation is ongoing, if the rate of denervation is balanced by the rate of reinnervation, fibrillations may not be recorded on NEE.

In addition to these inherent limitations, evaluating sensitivity and specificity of electrodiagnostic studies is complicated by the lack of a gold standard. For cervical radiculopathy, various criterion standards have been used, such as clinical, surgical, and radiologic findings, and account for a wide range of sensitivities, ranging from 50%[8] to 95%.[9] The false-positive rate of cervical MRI is somewhat lower, but still significant at 19%.[10] Electrodiagnostic studies and MRI agree in 60% of patients with symptoms suggestive of radiculopathy, and in 76% of cases when weakness is present. However, one study alone is positive in only 40% of cases.[11]

SENSORY NERVE CONDUCTION STUDIES

Abnormalities in sensory nerve action potentials (SNAP) are not part of the electrodiagnostic criteria of radiculopathy. However, their performance is necessary to rule out other potential diagnoses, such as peripheral polyneuropathy or entrapment mononeuropathy.[12] Sensory nerve parameters, including amplitude, distal latency, and nerve conduction velocity, are expected to be normal in radiculopathy.[13] If axon loss does not occur, symptoms of pain are mediated by C fibers, which are too small to be accessible by standard electrodiagnostic techniques. Even if axon loss does occur, the usual location of the lesion is proximal to the dorsal root ganglion and SNAPs, because they evaluate lesions distal to the dorsal root ganglia, do not show any abnormalities.[6] However, important exceptions to this dictum must be recognized. When pathology extends from the intraspinal space into the neural foramen and affects the dorsal root ganglion, as can happen with malignancy or infection, SNAP amplitude reduction occurs as a result of wallerian degeneration.[13] Additionally, SNAP amplitudes may be reduced when the dorsal root ganglion has an intraspinal location, making it vulnerable to lesions resulting from cervical spondylosis.

Nerve conduction studies in the electrodiagnostic evaluation of radiculopathy also evaluate for entrapment neuropathy. For example, the prevalence of carpal tunnel syndrome in patients with cervical radiculopathy has been estimated at 22.1%,[14] which is significantly greater than estimates for the general population (0.52% for men and 1.49% for women).[15] The double crush hypothesis was put forth in 1973 by Upton and McComas[16] and proposes that a proximal lesion along an axon, such as that caused by radiculopathy, predisposes it to injury at a more distal site. However, later studies do not reveal any correlation between the presence of cervical radiculopathy and abnormal median nerve conduction studies.[17–19] Another theory as to why carpal tunnel syndrome is more prevalent in patients with cervical radiculopathy is that both disorders have a common etiology, such as osteoarthritis, that can lead to both cervical foraminal and carpal tunnel stenosis.[14]

MOTOR NERVE CONDUCTION STUDIES

Compound muscle action potentials (CMAP) may be abnormal in the presence of a radiculopathy if axon loss is present. The amplitude of the CMAP can provide a semiquantitative measure of the number of axons supplying the muscle from which the recording was made.[20] However, the CMAP amplitude is not perfectly sensitive to the presence of a cervical radiculopathy. Significant reduction in CMAP amplitudes occurs with loss of approximately 50% of motor axons[13] and it is rare for this many nerve root fibers to degenerate.[6] Additionally, muscles typically have an overlapping nerve supply, allowing for redundancy even if individual nerve roots are compromised.

Another limitation of using CMAP to diagnose cervical radiculopathies is that the most commonly performed upper extremity studies are to the C8 and T1 innervated abductor pollicis brevis and the abductor digiti minimi. However, the most common cervical radiculopathies occur at C7 and C6,[6,21] and as such the most commonly performed upper extremity motor nerve conduction studies may be insensitive for the most common cervical radiculopathies.

LATE RESPONSES

Late responses are so named because their latency exceeds that of the more commonly studied M wave. One of the theoretical advantages to late responses is the ability to study proximal nerve segments, where the pathology of radiculopathy lies.

H-reflex

The H-reflex was first described by Hoffman in 1918,[22] and subsequently hypothesized by Magladery and coworkers[23] to be a monosynaptic reflex that assesses the afferent Ia sensory nerve and an efferent alpha motor nerve. However, other experimental studies have proposed that the pathways generating the H-reflex likely receive an oligosynaptic contribution.[24] In clinical practice, the H-reflex is most commonly obtained by stimulating the tibial nerve in the popliteal fossa and recording over the gastroc-soleus to assess the S1 nerve root. It may also be obtained by recording from the flexor carpi radialis (FCR)[25] in the forearm, and is obtainable in 90%[25] to 95%[26] of subjects. This test may be used in the electrodiagnosis of C6 and C7 radiculopathies, and remains normal in patients with C5 and C8 radiculopathies.[27] The sensitivities and specificities of the FCR H-reflex have been found to be 50% and 86% for C6 radiculopathy, and 75% and 86% for C7 radiculopathy.[28] The upper limit of normal latency is 21 milliseconds with 1.5 milliseconds of side-to-side variation.[22] The FCR H-reflex may be elicited by the technique described by Jabre,[25] in which the E-1 is placed over the belly of the FCR (one third of the distance between the medial epicondyle and radial styloid), the reference over the brachioradialis, and the ground between the stimulator and the E-1 electrode.

F wave

So named because they were originally recorded in the intrinsic foot muscles,[23] the F wave is a late response produced by supramaximal stimulation resulting in antidromic activation of motor neurons.[22] Latency is the parameter most frequently used in the evaluation of F waves.[22] Minimum latency is reported most commonly,[13] but mean F wave latencies may dilute measurement error and produce more consistent results.[29] Methods of eliciting the F wave from hand muscles[22] and also the FCR have been described.[30] When used to evaluate L5/S1 radiculopathy, the sensitivity of F wave abnormalities is impressively close to that of the NEE.[31,32] However, F wave abnormalities are less sensitive in detecting cervical radiculopathy. A study by Lo and colleagues[33] found that use of six different F wave parameters (minimal latency, chronodispersion, persistence, and right-left difference) yielded a sensitivity of 55% when using MRI as a gold standard. Additionally, the specificity of F waves may be limited by the "dilution" effect of latency abnormalities being hidden by the lengthy course of nerve fibers and, like H-reflexes, that abnormalities result from any pathology affecting proximal nerve segments in addition to radiculopathy.[6] An example of this is radial nerve conduction block causing abnormal F waves.[34]

EVOKED POTENTIALS

Evoked potentials are the responses of the central nervous system to external stimuli and somatosensory evoked potentials (SEP) occur as a result of stimulation of afferent peripheral nerve fibers.[35] The use of SEPs in the evaluation of radiculopathy remains controversial.[36] The most recent American Association of Neuromuscular and Electrodiagnostic Medicine (AANEM) guideline devoted to the subject indicates that SEPs may be helpful in cervical spondylosis when spinal cord compression is present, and that they may be more sensitive to sensory pathway involvement than clinical sensory testing.[35] The great strength of dermatomal SEPs is their ability to evaluate segmental level function throughout the neuraxis.[37] However, SEPs have several disadvantages.[13] Dermatomal SEPs cannot distinguish between the various causes of multiple-root disease, such as spinal stenosis or arachnoiditis, and are not believed to be useful for acute radiculopathy.[37–39] Amplitude measurements have too much normal variation to have clinical significance. Focal slowing in the root may be diluted by normal conduction in the remainder of the sensory pathway. Furthermore, SEPs evaluate the larger fiber tracts modulating proprioception and vibration, rather than the pain-mediating tracts that seem most commonly to elicit symptoms. These limitations, along with the technically demanding nature of the procedure, discourage their routine use.[13]

NEEDLE ELECTRODE EXAMINATION

The concept of using a myotomal distribution of abnormalities on NEE to localize a spinal segment was first reported in 1944[40] and is now a cornerstone of the electrodiagnostic evaluation of radiculopathy. Radiculopathy is suggested when abnormalities are noted in at least two muscles innervated by the same root, but different peripheral nerves, provided that muscles innervated by adjacent roots are normal.[6] Needle EMG evaluates for axonal loss, and reveals demyelination through reduced recruitment of motor units when conduction block is present.[6,13,41]

The NEE may also provide information about the chronicity of denervation. A study by Kraft[42] of 69 patients with traumatic peripheral nerve injury revealed that fibrillation amplitudes may be used to estimate time since nerve injury. The mean amplitude of fibrillations within 2 months after denervation was 612 μV, and decreased to less than 100 μV after 12 months. The same study found that reduction of fibrillation potential amplitudes also correlated with muscle fiber atrophy in a guinea pig model.[42] Another study evaluating the upper extremities of 173 patients with complete denervation of the biceps brachii because of brachial plexus injury revealed similar findings.[43] In this study, fibrillation amplitude within 2 months was 501 μV and showed decrease over time, but in contrast to Kraft's[42] study remained greater than 100 μV (262 μV) after 12 months. As noted in animal studies,[42] the reduction in fibrillation amplitude correlates with muscle fiber atrophy, and Type II muscle fiber atrophy is more rapid than Type I.

The most recent AANEM guidelines indicate that for evaluation of cervical radiculopathy, at least one muscle from each myotome C5 to T1 and the cervical paraspinal muscles should be studied.[12] However, the guidelines do not specify how many muscles should be examined. NEE can be uncomfortable to the patient, so studying the minimum number of required muscles is desirable. Additionally, not all radiculopathies are confirmable by EMG.[6] These include radiculopathies that are either exclusively sensory,[6] or in which the rate of denervation is balanced by the rate of reinnervation.[44] In these cases, electrodiagnostic abnormalities are not found regardless of how many muscles are studied.[44] Screening NEE was developed to minimize the number of studied muscles while maximizing the probability of detecting an electrodiagnostically confirmable radiculopathy.[44] A prior retrospective study[45] determined that screens involving seven muscles, along with cervical paraspinals, identify 93% to 98% of all electrodiagnostically confirmed cervical radiculopathies. However, in 2001, Dillingham and colleagues[46] determined that only six muscles along with cervical paraspinals still identified 94% to 99% of cervical radiculopathies, with additional muscles adding only minimal sensitivity. This study also recommends that if paraspinal muscles cannot be studied, eight limb muscles are necessary to detect greater than 92% of cervical radiculopathies. Of note, the study does not prescribe a specific set of muscles, just the number of muscles that must be studied. However, it does identify that a screen of paraspinals, deltoid, triceps, pronator teres, extensor digitorum communis, and abductor pollicus brevis yielded sensitivities of 99% using recruitment changes as diagnostic criteria and 83% using abnormal spontaneous activity.[46] If any of the screening muscles are abnormal, additional muscles may need to be studied to confirm the radiculopathy.[46]

Abnormalities on NEE may encompass any of a variety of neuropathic findings, such as polyphasia, reduced recruitment, increased insertional activity, complex repetitive discharges, or large-amplitude and long-duration motor unit action potentials (MUAP). With chronic denervation and subsequent reinnervation, the duration of MUAPs increases commensurate with the degree of collateral sprouting.[6,36] Unfortunately, reliably determining MUAP duration requires the quantitative evaluation of at least 20 motor units,[47] which is far too lengthy a procedure to recommend for clinical practice. Polyphasic MUAPs contain greater than four phases, and may indicate motor unit remodeling caused by chronic denervation and reinnervation.[6,36] Early studies[48,49] have indicated that isolated polyphasia may be the only finding in 35% to 75% of cases. However, using polyphasia as the sole diagnostic criterion for radiculopathy is problematic, because up to 20% of MUAPs in normal muscle may be polyphasic.[6,36] As with duration, differentiation of true polyphasia from "pseudopolyphasia" requires the use of a delay and trigger line,[50] which may not be done in routine NEE.

Spontaneous activity, such as fibrillations and positive sharp waves, may be a more reliable indicator than the motor unit remodeling parameters described previously. However, with these certain pitfalls must be recognized. Conventionally, spontaneous activity occurring after acute radiculopathy is thought to appear first in the paraspinals in approximately 1 week, and to manifest in more distal limb muscles in several weeks.[6,36] As such, an improperly timed study may miss abnormalities. However, recent prospective evidence has challenged this theory, and indicates no correlation between paraspinal spontaneous activity and symptom duration in both the cervical and lumbar spine.[51]

SEGMENTAL LOCALIZATION

In 50 patients with surgically proved single-root lesions, the following patterns of positive sharp waves or fibrillations on NEE emerged[52]:

- C5 radiculopathy: The infraspinatus, supraspinatus, biceps, deltoid, and brachioradialis showed approximately equal incidences of spontaneous activity.
- C7 radiculopathy: The FCR, anconeus, pronator teres, and triceps were most frequently affected.
- C8 radiculopathy: Most typically affected the first dorsal interosseus, extensor indicus proprius, and abductor digiti minimi, and less frequently the flexor pollicis longus and abductor pollicis brevis.
- C6 radiculopathy: Produces the most variable pattern of abnormalities and can mimic either the findings of C5 radiculopathy with the addition of pronator teres, or the findings of a C7 radiculopathy.

THE PARASPINAL MUSCLES

Abnormalities of the paraspinal muscles are considered to localize a lesion proximal to the plexus.[53] However, spontaneous activity in the paraspinals may be found in a variety of conditions, including diabetes[6]; minor trauma, such as lumbar puncture[54];

posterior approach spinal surgery[55]; and in up to 4% of asymptomatic, healthy people.[56] Notably, paraspinal abnormalities are not part of the electrodiagnostic criteria of radiculopathy[12]; however, sensitivity and specificity are improved if cervical paraspinals are included in the screen.[44] Therefore, the evaluation of paraspinal abnormalities must be made in light of the remainder of the electrodiagnostic findings and in corroboration with the history and physical examination. In the author's experience, cervical paraspinal abnormalities may only be appreciated in relatively small segmental regions of deep paramedian muscle fibers. Examination is frequently easier if special attention is given to patient positioning in the side-lying position with neck flexion and head support to keep the spine in midline.

OUTCOMES

Electrodiagnostic confirmation of a radiculopathy may have important implications when surgery is contemplated. In a relatively small sample size study, Alrawi and colleagues[57] demonstrated that patients with electrodiagnostically confirmed cervical radiculopathy had improved outcomes following diskectomy and anterior fusion compared with postoperative patients who did not have electrophysiologic evidence of radiculopathy. Conversely, when visual analog scales were used as an outcome measure, the absence of electrodiagnostic confirmation was correlated with poor postoperative results.[58]

SUMMARY

Radiculopathy can be a challenging diagnosis resulting from multiple etiologies. Although imaging may elucidate the structural causes of radiculopathy, imaging cannot pinpoint the cause of radiculopathy when either multiple structural abnormalities are present, or when radiculopathy results from nonstructural causes. Electrodiagnosis provides a means of functional assessment of the nerve root, and may also provide prognostic information regarding functional outcomes of patients with radiculopathy.

REFERENCES

1. Lauder TD, Dillingham TR, Andary M, et al. Predicting electrodiagnostic outcome in patients with upper limb symptoms: are the history and physical examination helpful? Arch Phys Med Rehabil 2000;81:436–41.
2. Uysal II, Seker M, Karabulut AK, et al. Brachial plexus variations in human fetuses. Neurosurgery 2003;53:676–84.
3. Loukas M, Lewis RG Jr, Wartman CT. T2 contributions to the brachial plexus. Neurosurgery 2007;60:S13–8.
4. Pellerin M, Kimball Z, Tubbs RS, et al. The prefixed and postfixed brachial plexus: a review with surgical implications. Surg Radiol Anat 2010;32:251–60.
5. Johnson EO, Vekris M, Demesticha T, et al. Neuroanatomy of the brachial plexus: normal and variant anatomy of its formation. Surg Radiol Anat 2010;32:291–7.
6. Wilbourn AJ, Aminoff MJ. AAEM Minimonograph 32: the electrodiagnostic examination in patients with radiculopathies. Muscle Nerve 1998;21:1612–31.
7. Waylonis GW. Electromyographic findings in chronic cervical radicular symptoms. Arch Phys Med Rehabil 1968;49:407–12.
8. Yiannikas C, Shahani BT, Young RR. Short-latency somatosensory-evoked potentials from radial, median, ulnar, and peroneal nerve stimulation in the assessment of cervical spondylosis. Arch Neurol 1986;43:1264–71.

9. Tackman W, Radu EW. Observations of the application of electrophysiological methods in the diagnosis of cervical root compressions. Eur Neurol 1983;22: 397–404.

10. Boden SD, McCowin PR, Davis DO, et al. Abnormal magnetic-resonance scans of the cervical spine in asymptomatic subjects. J Bone Joint Surg Am 1990;72: 1178–84.

11. Nardin RA, Patel MR, Gudas TF, et al. Electromyography and magnetic resonance imaging in the evaluation of radiculopathy. Muscle Nerve 1999;22:151–5.

12. American Association of Electrodiagnostic Medicine. Practice parameter for needle electromyographic evaluation of patients with suspected cervical radiculopathy: summary statement. Muscle Nerve 1999;22(Suppl 8):S209–11.

13. Levin KH. Electrodiagnostic approach to the patient with suspected radiculopathy. Neurol Clin 2002;20:397–421.

14. Richardson JK, Forman GM, Riley B. An electrophysiological exploration of the double crush hypothesis. Muscle Nerve 1999;22:71–7.

15. Stevens JC, Sun S, Beard CM, et al. Carpal tunnel syndrome in Rochester, Minnesota, 1961 to 1980. Neurology 1988;38(1):134–8.

16. Upton AR, McComas AJ. The double crush in nerve entrapment syndromes. Lancet 1973;2:359–62.

17. Kwon HK, Hwang M, Yoon DW. Frequency and severity of carpal tunnel syndrome according to level of cervical radiculopathy: double crush syndrome? Clin Neurophysiol 2006;117:1256–9.

18. Frith RW, Litchy WJ. Electrophysiologic abnormalities of peripheral nerves in patients with cervical radiculopathy. Muscle Nerve 1985;8:613.

19. Morgan G, Wilbourn AJ. Cervical radiculopathy and coexisting distal entrapment neuropathies: double crush syndrome? Neurology 1998;50:78–83.

20. Wilbourn AJ. AAEE case report #12: common peroneal mononeuropathy at the fibular head. Muscle Nerve 1986;9:825–36.

21. Radhakrishnan K, Litchy WJ, O'Fallon WM, et al. Epidemiology of cervical radiculopathy. A population-based study from Rochester, Minnesota, 1976 through 1990. Brain 1994;117:325–35.

22. Fisher MA. H reflexes and F waves, fundamentals, normal and abnormal patterns. Neurol Clin 2002;20:339–60.

23. Magladery JW, Teasdall RD, Magladery JW. Electrophysiological studies of nerve and reflex activity in normal man. IV. The two-neurone reflex and identification of certain action potentials from spinal roots and cord. Bull Johns Hopkins Hosp 1951;88(6):499–519.

24. Burke D, Gandevia SC, McKeon B. Monosynaptic and oligosynaptic contributions to the human ankle jerk and H-reflex. J Neurophysiol 1984;52(3):435–48.

25. Jabre JF. Surface recording of the H-reflex of the flexor carpi radialis. Muscle Nerve 1981;4:435–8.

26. Christie AD, Inglis JG, Boucher JP, et al. Reliability of the FCR H-reflex. J Clin Neurophysiol 2005;22(3):204–9.

27. Schimsheimer RJ, Ongerboer de Visser BW, Kemp B. The flexor carpi radialis H-reflex in lesions of the sixth and seventh cervical nerve roots. J Neurol Neurosurg Psychiatr 1985;48:445–9.

28. Eliaspour D, Sanati E, Hedayati Moqadam MR, et al. Utility of flexor carpi radialis H-reflex in diagnosis of cervical radiculopathy. J Clin Neurophysiol 2009;26(6):458–60.

29. Panayiotoupoulos CP, Chroni E. F-waves in clinical neurophysiology: a review, methodological issues and overall value in peripheral neuropathies. Electroencephalogr Clin Neurophysiol 1996;101:365–74.

30. Marchini C, Marinig R, Bergonzi P. Median nerve F-wave study derived by flexor carpi radialis. Electromyogr Clin Neurophysiol 1998;38(8):451–3.
31. Toyokura M, Murakami K. F-wave study in patients with lumbosacral radiculopathies. Electromyogr Clin Neurophysiol 1997;37(1):19–26.
32. Scelsa SN, Herskovitz S, Berger AR. The diagnostic utility of F waves in L5/S1 radiculopathy. Muscle Nerve 1995;18(12):1496–7.
33. Lo YL, Chan LL, Leoh T, et al. Diagnostic utility of F waves in cervical radiculopathy: electrophysiological and magnetic resonance imaging correlation. Clin Neurol Neurosurg 2008;110(1):58–61.
34. Papathanasiou E, Kleopa KA, Pantzaris M. Unobtainable radial nerve F-waves in a case of radial nerve conduction block. Electromyogr Clin Neurophysiol 2004; 44(8):451–4.
35. American Association of Electrodiagnostic Medicine. Somatosensory evoked potentials: clinical uses. Muscle Nerve 1999;22(Suppl 8):S111–8.
36. Fisher MA. Electrophysiology of radiculopathies. Clin Neurophysiol 2002;113: 317–35.
37. Storm SA, Kraft GH. The clinical use of dermatomal somatosensory evoked potentials in lumbosacral spinal stenosis. Phys Med Rehabil Clin N Am 2004; 15:107–15.
38. Kraft GH. Dermatomal somatosensory-evoked potentials in the evaluation of lumbosacral spinal stenosis. Phys Med Rehabil Clin N Am 2003;14:71–5.
39. Kraft GH. A physiological approach to the evaluation of lumbosacral spinal stenosis. Phys Med Rehabil Clin N Am 1998;9(2):381–9.
40. Hoefer PF, Guttman SA. Electromyography as a method for determination of level of lesions in the spinal cord. Arch Neurol Psychiatr 1944;51(5):415–22.
41. Tsao B. The electrodiagnosis of cervical and lumbosacral radiculopathy. Neurol Clin 2007;25:473–94.
42. Kraft GH. Fibrillation potential amplitude and muscle atrophy following peripheral nerve injury. Muscle Nerve 1990;13:814–21.
43. Jiang GL, Zhang LY, Shen LY, et al. Fibrillation potential amplitude to quantitatively assess denervation muscle atrophy. Neuromuscul Disord 2000;10:85–91.
44. Dillingham TR, Lauder TD, Andary M, et al. Identifying lumbosacral radiculopathies: an optimal electromyographic screen. Am J Phys Med Rehabil 2000;79: 496–503.
45. Lauder TD, Dillingham TR. The cervical radiculopathy screen: optimizing the number of muscles studied. Muscle Nerve 1996;19:662–5.
46. Dillingham TR, Lauder TD, Andary M, et al. Identification of cervical radiculopathies: optimizing the electromyographic screen. Am J Phys Med Rehabil 2001; 80(84–91):84.
47. Buchthal F, Pinell P, Rosenfalck P. Action potential parameters in normal human muscle and their physiological determinants. Acta Physiol Scand 1954;32(2/3): 219–29.
48. Crane CR, Krusen EM. Significance of polyphasic potentials in the diagnosis of cervical root involvement. Arch Phys Med Rehabil 1968;49:403–6.
49. LaJoie WJ. Nerve root compression: correlation of electromyographic, myelographic, and surgical findings. Arch Phys Med Rehabil 1972;53:390–2.
50. Dumitru D, Amato AA, Zwarts M, editors. Electrodiagnostic medicine. 2nd edition. Philadelphia: Hanley & Belfus; 2002.
51. Dillingham TR, Pezzin LE, Lauder TD, et al. Symptom duration and spontaneous activity in lumbosacral radiculopathy. Am J Phys Med Rehabil 2000;79(2): 124–32.

52. Levin KH, Maggiano HJ, Wilbourn AJ. Cervical radiculopathies: comparison of surgical and EMG localization of single-root lesions. Neurology 1996;46(4): 1022–5.
53. Woods WW, Shea PA. The value of electromyography in neurology and neurosurgery. J Neurosurg 1951;8(6):595–607.
54. Danner R. Occurrence of transient positive sharp wave like activity in the paraspinal muscles following lumbar puncture. Electromyogr Clin Neurophysiol 1982;22:149–54.
55. Johnson EW, Burkhart JA, Eart WC. Electromyography in postlaminectomy patients. Arch Phys Med Rehabil 1972;53:407–9.
56. Dumitru D, Diaz CA, King JC. Prevalence of denervation in paraspinal and foot intrinsic musculature. Am J Phys Med Rehabil 2001;80:482–90.
57. Alrawi MF, Khalil NM, Mitchell P, et al. The value of neurophysiological and imaging studies in predicting outcome in the surgical treatment of cervical radiculopathy. Eur Spine J 2007;16(4):495–500.
58. Tullberg T, Svanborg E, Isaccsson J, et al. A preoperative and postoperative study of the accuracy and value of electrodiagnosis in patients with lumbosacral disc herniation. Spine (Phila Pa 1976) 1993;18(7):837–42.

Cervical Radiculopathy

Steve H. Yoon, MD

KEYWORDS

• Cervical • Radiculopathy • Neck • Pain

With regards to spinal disorders, neck pain is one of the most common presenting symptoms, only second to low back pain. It is more often spontaneous in onset without having a specific inciting event.[1] When pain radiates down the arm and is associated with sensory and motor disturbances, cervical radiculopathy is suspected. Cervical radiculopathy occurs when a nerve root is compressed or irritated, causing associated sensory, motor, or reflex changes in the affected nerve root distribution.[2] It is a substantial cause of disability and morbidity and occurs in both genders, typically during the middle ages.[3]

EPIDEMIOLOGY

A population-based study from Rochester, Minn., found the annual age-adjusted incidence of cervical radiculopathy to be 83 cases per 100,000 persons. The annual incidence rate was higher for men, with a rate of 107 cases per 100,000 persons for men and 63 cases per 100,000 persons for women. The ages ranged from 13 to 91 years, with the peak incidence occurring at 50 to 54 years of age in both genders. In this study, either spondylosis, disk protrusion, or both were involved in nearly 70% of the cases.[4,5]

ANATOMY

There are a total of 8 cervical nerve roots, each exiting above the vertebrae of the same numeric designation, with the exception of C8, which exits above the T1 vertebrae. The neural foramina through the nerve roots exit are bordered anteromedially by the uncovertebral joint, posterolaterally by the facet joint, superiorly by the pedicle of the vertebral body above, and inferiorly by the pedicle of the vertebral body below. For example, the C6 nerve root exits through the C5-C6 neural foramen formed by the C5 and C6 vertebral bodies and disk.

PATHOPHYSIOLOGY

The three most common ways that compress or irritate an exiting nerve root include: herniation of a disc posterolaterally, degeneration of a disc causing decreased height

The author has nothing to disclose.
Kerlan-Jobe Orthopaedic Clinic, 6801 Park Terrace, Los Angeles, CA 90405, USA
E-mail address: steve.yoon@kerlanjobe.com

of the neural foramen, and cervical spondylosis, which can occur at the vertebral body, uncovertebral joint, or facet joint.[2] Cervical degenerative changes have been shown to occur in those over 40 years old.[6,7] The progressive loss of the disc's viscoelastic properties can lead to loss of disc height and vertebral end plate stress. As a result, osteophytes are formed, which serve to increase the overall surface area and counterbalance the increased stress.[7] This decrease in disc height can also cause increased joint stress, leading to hypertrophy of the uncovertebral and facet joints as arthritic changes occur. Both formation of osteophytes and hypertrophied joints, known collectively as cervical spondylosis, can contribute to an obstructive occlusion of the neural foramen leading to impingement. With regards to disc herniations, the posterior longitudinal ligament is oftentimes weaker than its anterior counterpart and thus, with excess pressure applied to the cervical disc, a herniation can occur posteriorly. When this herniation is broad enough or extends laterally into the intervertebral foramen, an occlusion may occur.[7]

The exact pathogenesis of radicular pain remains unclear, but it is thought that compression alone may not always be enough to cause pain, and that an inflammatory chemical component is needed. It has been found that chemical mediators involved in the inflammatory process are released from sensory neurons and intervertebral disc tissues, contributing to the occurrence of pain.[8] Further studies have found that compression of the dorsal root ganglion alone can cause an inflammatory response by causing prolonged cell body discharges. In addition, increased permeability of the membrane of the dorsal root ganglion with respects to its surrounding nerve root membrane is also hypothesized to be a potential source for radicular pain.[9]

Compromise of the neural foramen resulting in impingement of the exiting nerve root may also result in impairment of the blood supply to the nerve itself. Radicular arteries within the dural root sleeve as well as venous flow may be inhibited, causing spasm and ultimately decreased perfusion to the nerve.[7,10] Insult to the nerve root also can result in increased permeability of the intrinsic blood vessels, causing edema to occur within the nerve root itself. This chronic edema and fibrosis can eventually increase the nerve's membrane threshold and increase sensitivity to pain.[9,11]

Overall, in the younger population, cervical radiculopathy is often attributed to a disc herniation or an acute injury causing foraminal stenosis. Cervical spondylosis contributing to foraminal narrowing is usually observed in an older population.[12] One study showed that in 70% to 75% of cases, foraminal encroachment was responsible for cervical radiculopathy versus 20% to 25% of cases due to disk herniation.[4] The C7 nerve root is the most commonly affected followed by C6, C8, and C5 in descending order of incidence.[2,12]

CLINICAL PRESENTATION

Patients typically present with neck pain radiating to the upper extremity. The distribution of the radiating pain depends on the cervical levels that are involved. Typically, pain is distributed in a myotomal pattern but can also involve surrounding areas, including the suboccipital, scapular, and, rarely, chest wall regions.[2] Sensory symptoms such as numbness and tingling usually occur in a dermatomal pattern.[13,14] A subset of patients will present with weakness alone without any significant pain or sensory symptoms. In this case, proper investigation is needed to assess whether an alternative diagnosis is present, including the presence of a myelopathy. Cervical myelopathy may present with deficits such as decreased sensation in the hands or fine motor skills, as well as poor balance and bowel and bladder dysfunction.[2] The latter deficits are typically not found in cervical radiculopathy and should be investigated thoroughly. The timing of the presenting symptoms may also help distinguish the pathologic etiology. An acute or subacute presentation may be related to a disc herniation, whereas a slow and insidious presentation may be due to cervical spondylosis.[15]

PHYSICAL EXAMINATION

Observation of the patient's movements specific to the cervical spine as well as generalized movements such as gait and posture will help fully assess the patient. Detection of muscle atrophy in the shoulder girdle and upper extremities should be noted. Palpation of the cervical spine and surrounding muscles will help detect any deformities such as loss of lordosis, tenderness, or muscle spasms. Cervical spine range of motion should be fully assessed to determine limitations. In addition, lateral rotation or bending towards the affected side may occlude the neural foramen and reproduce symptoms.[2]

Assessment for weakness, sensory changes, and diminished reflexes is useful for the detection and isolation of the nerve roots involved in a cervical radiculopathy (**Table 1**). Profound myotomal weakness is rare, as most muscles have innervations from at least 2 nerve roots. Consideration for polyneuropathy including polyradiculopathy or brachial plexopathy should be given. Dermatomal changes will typically be found in the distal dermatome distribution. Gait and lower extremity strength testing can help determine whether a myelopathy is present. Also, upper motor neuron signs should be documented, including Hoffman sign, hyper-reflexia, Babinski response, and clonus. Provocative maneuvers can also be performed. Both Spurling and Scoville[16] described a provocative maneuver in which the patient's head was rotated toward the suspected side and, with applied downward pressure; the head was laterally bent towards that side. A positive test occurs with reproduction of the patient's radicular symptoms. The Spurling test has been shown to have a specificity of 93% and sensitivity of 30% in detecting cervical radiculopathy, indicating its use as a confirmative examination and not necessarily for screening.[12,17,18] Other tests that can be conducted include the shoulder abduction test, neck distraction test, and Valsalva maneuver test, all of which have less accuracy and reliability.

Table 1
Cervical nerve root associations on physical examination

Nerve Root	Pain Distribution	Motor	Sensory	Reflex
C4	Lower neck, trapezius	None	Cape distribution (lower neck and shoulder girdle)	None
C5	Neck, medial scapula, shoulder, lateral arm	Shoulder abduction, elbow flexion	Lateral upper arm	Biceps
C6	Neck, lateral forearm, first and second digit	Elbow flexion, wrist extension	Lateral forearm, first and second digit	Brachioradialis
C7	Neck, medial scapula, dorsal forearm, third digit	Elbow extension, wrist flexion	Dorsal forearm, third digit	Triceps
C8	Neck, medial forearm, fifth digit	Finger flexors, finger abduction and adduction	Medial forearm, fourth and fifth digit	None

Adapted from Polston DW. Cervical radiculopathy. Neurol Clin 2007;25:373–85; with permission.

DIAGNOSTIC EVALUATION
Laboratory Studies

Laboratory studies are not initially recommended unless an infectious etiology is suspected. Screening tests for acute-phase proteins such as C-reactive proteins or erythrocyte sedimentation rate are not sensitive or specific enough to provide any additional diagnostic value.

Imaging

Radiographic imaging of the cervical spine is an essential tool in the diagnosis of cervical radiculopathy. The American College of Radiology recommends the use of plain radiographs as the initial step in the evaluation of patients with neck pain.[19] Conventional radiographs do have their limitations, as they cannot detect disc herniations or nerve root compressions. However, visualization of osteophytes into the intervertebral foramen as well as other visual deformities can help determine whether further imaging is necessary. Magnetic resonance imaging (MRI) is the diagnostic test of choice when investigating the presence of cervical radiculopathy. The ability to differentiate between contrasting tissues, including intervertebral discs and nerve roots, allows the ability to detect abnormalities as well as identification of the particular level involved.[7,15] Attention must be made to correlate MRI findings with the patient's symptoms and physical findings as spondylotic changes are normally seen in adults and can be present in asymptomatic patients as well.[6] Computed tomography (CT) scans are able to accurately identify pertinent spondylotic changes such as foraminal encroachment, spur formations, facet arthropathy, and ossification of ligaments.[14] Intrathecal administration of contrast can also be used to assist in the identification of root or cord compression. For those with cardiac pacemakers or stainless steel hardware in the cervical spine, CT scan is the preferred imaging test of choice.

Electrodiagnostic Studies

Needle electromyography (EMG) and nerve conduction studies (NCS) can assist the clinician in differentiating possible causes of the patient's neuropathic symptoms (**Box 1**). Nerve conduction studies can assess amplitude, distal latency, and conduction velocity of nerves to determine the extent of axon loss and myelination. In addition, needle EMG testing of the muscles can detect abnormalities such as denervation and reinnervation potentials and analyze motor unit characteristics. This information can help determine the severity, extent, and chronicity of denervation.[15] Correlation with EMG and nerve conduction findings with the history, physical examination findings, and diagnostic imaging can provide enough comprehensive information to determine whether a cervical radiculopathy likely exists. Needle EMG can be sensitive but should be performed after a period of 18 to 21 days from the initial onset of injury, as denervation potentials such as positive sharp waves and fibrillations may not be present prior to this time period. With this said, normal EMG results after the 18- to 21- day period still do not exclude the presence of a cervical radiculopathy.

TREATMENT

Treatment options vary according to the acuity and severity of the patient's signs and symptoms. The goal is to alleviate the patient's symptoms and prevent any further deterioration. Conservative nonoperative treatments should be initially considered. Some patients may benefit from further education regarding cervical radiculopathy; however, a systematic review examining this showed that education did not benefit the treatment of isolated neck or radicular pain.[5,20] Most conservative treatments

Box 1
Common differential diagnosis for cervical radiculopathy
Brachial plexitis
Cardiac pain
Cervical myelopathy
Cervical disc injury
Cervical facet syndrome
Complex regional pain syndrome
Herpes zoster
Intraspinal and extraspinal tumors
Nerve entrapment syndromes
Parsonage-Turner syndrome
Pancoast syndrome
Rotator cuff injury
Thoracic outlet syndrome
Vasculitis

commonly prescribed today have not been rigorously examined in randomized, placebo-controlled trials, and as such, many recommendations are based on case reports and anecdotal evidence.[14]

Pharmacotherapy

Analgesic medications such as nonsteroidal anti-inflammatory drugs (NSAIDs) are often used as first-line therapy for cervical radiculopathy. Opioids are also used in the initial stages of treatment. A systematic review and meta-analysis nonspecific to cervical radiculopathy showed that opioids may be effective in the treatment of neuropathic pain up to 8 weeks of duration.[21] There is insufficient evidence to suggest benefit of opioids beyond 8 weeks.[5] During acute stages of a cervical radiculopathy, some practitioners may also utilize oral steroids as a stronger form of anti-inflammatory treatment. This may be given either as a prepackaged dose pack or as a dose equivalent to 1 mg/kg of body weight daily and tapered approximately 10 mg every day. This type of oral steroid prescribing is due to anecdotal evidence and is not supported by any high-quality studies showing benefit.[22] Muscle relaxants, antidepressants, and anticonvulsants all also have a role in the treatment of cervical radiculopathy. Muscle relaxants work on alleviating muscle tension around the affected site, and certain antidepressants (tricyclics and selective serotonin reuptake inhibitors) and anticonvulsants such as Gabapentin work through various mechanisms to provide neuropathic related pain relief.

Physical Therapy

Physical therapy is often prescribed, as it has been shown to provide some relief for patients, although currently there are no evidence-based quality studies that have shown any long-lasting benefit with this form of treatment alone.[23] Gentle range-of-motion and cervical stabilization exercises can be initiated along with passive treatments such as ice, heat, and electrical stimulation. As the patient progresses, strengthening exercises can be increased, and a home exercise program can be tailored to each individual.

Immobilization

The use of a soft or hard cervical collar has been recommended for short-term use only for acute cervical radiculopathy. Typically, a time frame of less than 2 weeks is recommended. There is no evidence to date suggesting that a cervical collar can alter the course or intensity of the disease process.[5,24] Use of a cervical pillow has also been mentioned as providing symptomatic relief; however, more data are needed to further assess this mode of treatment.[14]

Traction

Traction is the administration of a distracting force to the cervical spine in order to separate the cervical segments and provide relief to the compressed nerve roots. Numerous studies have evaluated the intricacies of this treatment, including duration, positioning, and type of traction device. A systematic review evaluating the literature was not able to draw any conclusions due to the lack of available quality data.[25]

Epidural Injections

Favorable outcomes have been reported in the literature to support the use of epidural corticosteroid injections for the treatment of cervical radiculopathy using either an interlaminar or transforaminal approach. Short-term pain relief has been documented for the treatment of cervical radicular symptoms,[26] while in another study, as many as 60% of patients reported long-term relief of their neck and radicular symptoms.[27] The literature does not provide any conclusive evidence to support interlaminar versus transforaminal approaches. However, serious neurologic complications (infarction of spinal cord, brainstem, or brain) have been documented, especially using the transforaminal approach.

Surgery

Surgical fixation may be an option for patients with cervical radiculopathy if nonoperative treatments do not provide adequate relief. If this is the case, often patients will be considered for surgery if they continue to display persistent signs and symptoms that last greater than 6 weeks and have appropriate correlation with cervical nerve root compression on imaging. In addition, motor deficits that continue to be present as well as progression of neurologic deficits from the initial of onset may also warrant evaluation for surgery.

REFERENCES

1. Devereaux M. Neck pain. Med Clin North Am 2009;93:273–84.
2. Cohen I, Jouve C. Cervical radiculopathy. In: Frontera WR, Silver JK, Rizzo TD Jr, editors. Frontera: essentials of physical medicine and rehabilitation. Philadelphia: Saunders Elsevier; 2008. p. 17–22.
3. Rubinstein SM, Pool JJ, van Tulder MW, et al. A systematic review of the diagnostic accuracy of provocative tests of the neck for diagnosing cervical radiculopathy. Eur Spine J 2007;16:307–19.
4. Radhakrishan K, Litchy WJ, O'Fallon WM, et al. Epidemiology of cervical radiculopathy: a population-based study from Rochester, Minnesota, 1976 through 1990. Brain 1994;117:325–35.

5. Eubanks JD. Cervical radiculopathy: nonoperative management of neck pain and radicular symptoms. Am Fam Physician 2010;81(1):33–40.
6. Boden SD, McCowin PR, Davis DO, et al. Abnormal magnetic resonance scans of the cervical spine in asymptomatic subjects. J Bone Joint Surg 1990;72A: 1178–84.
7. Manifold SG, McCann PD. Cervical radiculitis and shoulder disorders. Clin Orthop Relat Res 1999;368:105–13.
8. Chabot MC, Montgomery DM. The pathophysiology of axial and radicular neck pain. Semin Spine Surg 1995;7:2–8.
9. Rao R. Neck pain, cervical radiculopathy, and cervical myelopathy. J Bone Joint Surg Am 2002;84A(10):1872–81.
10. Hoff JT, Papadopoulos SM. Cervical disc disease and cervical spondylosis. In: Wilkins RH, Rengachary SS, editors. Neurosurgery. 2nd edition. New York: McGraw-Hill; 1985. p. 3765–74.
11. Cooper RG, Freemont AJ, Hoyland JA, et al. Herniated intervertebral disc-associated periradicular fibrosis and vascular abnormalities occur without inflammatory cell infiltration. Spine 1995;20:591–8.
12. Malanga GA. The diagnosis and treatment of cervical radiculopathy. Med Sci Sports Exerc 1997;29:S236–45.
13. Slipman CW, Plastaras CT, Palmitier RA, et al. Symptom provocation of fluoroscopically guided cervical nerve root stimulation: are dynatomal maps identical to dermatomal maps? Spine 1998;23:2235–42.
14. Carette S, Fehlings M. Cervical radiculopathy. N Engl J Med 2005;353:392–9.
15. Polston DW. Cervical radiculopathy. Neurol Clin 2007;25:373–85.
16. Spurling RG, Scoville WB. Lateral rupture of the cervical intervertebral discs: a common cause of shoulder and arm pain. Surg Gynecol Obstet 1944;78: 350–8.
17. Tong HC, Haig AJ, Yamakawa K. The Spurling test and cervical radiculopathy. Spine (Phila Pa 1976) 2002;27(2):156–9.
18. Nordin M, Carragee EJ, Hogg-Johnson S, et al, for the Bone and Joint Decade 2000–2010 Task Force on Neck Pain and Its Associated Disorders. Assessment of neck pain and its associated disorders: results of the Bone and Joint Decade 2000–2010 Task Force on Neck Pain and Its Associated Disorders. Spine 2008; 33(Suppl 4):S101–22.
19. Mink JH, Gordon RE, Deutsch AL. The cervical spine: radiologist's perspective. Phys Med Rehabil Clin N Am 2003;14:493–548.
20. Haines T, Gross A, Burnie SJ, et al. Patient education for neck pain with or without radiculopathy. Cochrane Database Syst Rev 2009;1:CD005106.
21. Eisenberg E, McNicol ED, Carr DB. Efficacy and safety of opioid agonists in the treatment of neuropathic pain of nonmalignant origin: systematic review and meta-analysis of randomized controlled trials. JAMA 2005;293(24):3043–52.
22. Rhee JM, Yoon T, Riew KD. Cervical radiculopathy. J Am Acad Orthop Surg 2007; 15(8):486–94.
23. Cleland JA, Whitman JM, Fritz JM, et al. Manual physical therapy, cervical traction, and strengthening exercises in patients with cervical radiculopathy: a case series. J Orthop Sports Phys Ther 2005;35:802–11.
24. Levine MJ, Albert TJ, Smith MD. Cervical radiculopathy: diagnosis and nonoperative management. J Am Acad Orthop Surg 1996;4(6):305–16.
25. Van der Heijden GJ, Beurskens AJ, Koes BW, et al. The efficacy of traction for back and neck pain: a systematic, blinded review of randomized clinical trial methods. Phys Ther 1995;75:93–104.

26. Carragee EJ, Hurwitz EL, Cheng I, et al. Treatment of neck pain: injections and surgical interventions: results of the Bone and Joint Decade 2000–2010 Task Force on Neck Pain and Its Associated Disorders. Spine 2008;33(4): S153–69.

27. Slipman CW, Lipetz JS, Jackson HB, et al. Therapeutic selective nerve root block in the nonsurgical treatment of atraumatic cervical spondylotic radicular pain: a retrospective analysis with independent clinical review. Arch Phys Med Rehabil 2000;81:741–6.

Cervical Facet-Mediated Pain

Alfred C. Gellhorn, MD[a,b,*]

KEYWORDS

• Cervical • Neck • Pain • Facet • Zygapophyseal • Whiplash

The cervical zygapophyseal joints, or facet joints, have long been implicated as a source of neck pain. This article examines the epidemiology of pain arising from these joints, as well as relevant anatomy and histology. An emphasis on clinical findings, examination, and imaging are presented, as well as a focus on whiplash-associated pain, in which the facet joints are frequently implicated as the source of pain.

A semantic and lexical issue must be briefly discussed before commencement, however. The terms zygapophyseal joint and facet joint are often used interchangeably in the medical literature to name these joints, although the terms are not technically synonymous. The term *zygapophysis*, first used in 1854,[1] and etymologically formed from the Greek for yoke and offshoot, refers specifically to the lateral process on the neural arch of a vertebra that articulates with the corresponding process of the next vertebra. The term *facet* is less specific, and is defined in the Oxford English Dictionary as a small, clearly delimited smooth area, especially an articular surface, on a vertebra or other bone.[2] While *zygapophyseal* is more anatomically specific and may therefore be felt to be preferable in reference to this structure, the term *facet* appears to have greater acceptance based on usage in published studies. A recent PubMed search revealed a total of 3109 articles referring to this joint, of which 2737 (88%) referred to the facet joint exclusively, and 846 (27%) referred to the zygapophyseal joint exclusively. Fifteen percent of studies hedged and use both naming conventions. Sober evaluation of these findings reveals the uncomfortable truth that searching the literature for studies concerning this structure using only one or the other naming convention will miss a significant portion of the available evidence. In this article, the terms are used interchangeably, reflecting an appreciation for both the anatomic specificity of this structure, and the unequivocal preference for a more colloquial term among those who have studied and written about it.

The author has nothing to disclose.
[a] Department of Rehabilitation Medicine, University of Washington, Box 354740, 4245 Roosevelt Way NE, Seattle, WA 98105, USA
[b] Department of Orthopedics and Sports Medicine, University of Washington, Box 354740, 4245 Roosevelt Way NE, Seattle, WA 98105, USA
* Department of Rehabilitation Medicine, University of Washington, Box 354740, 4245 Roosevelt Way NE, Seattle, WA 98105.
E-mail address: gellhorn@uw.edu

Phys Med Rehabil Clin N Am 22 (2011) 447–458
doi:10.1016/j.pmr.2011.02.006
1047-9651/11/$ – see front matter © 2011 Elsevier Inc. All rights reserved.
pmr.theclinics.com

EPIDEMIOLOGY OF FACET-MEDIATED NECK PAIN

Neck pain is common, and most people can expect to have some degree of neck pain at some point in their life.[3] Estimates of neck pain prevalence rates vary by study and patient population. A recent systematic review on the prevalence of neck pain in the general population considered 54 studies and found a 12-month prevalence range of 12% to 72%. However, most estimates of 12-month prevalence fell between 30% and 50%, with activity-limiting pain in 1.7% to 11.5%.[4] Prevalence of neck pain in workers was found to be similar to those in the general population, with 12-month prevalence rates between 27% in Norway to 48% in Quebec, Canada. Between 11% and 14% of workers were limited in their activities because of neck pain each year.[5] Another study of office workers found that neck pain had the highest prevalence among all musculoskeletal complaints, at 42%.[6]

Studies attempting to determine the proportion of neck pain related to the facet joints have focused more on patient populations with chronic pain than those with acute pain, largely because precise and accurate determination of the source of neck pain is based on anesthetic injections, the risks of which limit their use in the setting of acute and self-limited symptoms. However, in cases of chronic axial neck pain, the cervical facet joints have been reported to be the source of pain in between 25% to 66% of cases.[7] In cases of traumatically induced chronic neck pain, facet involvement has been found in 50% to 60% of cases.[8] Some studies suggest that traumatically induced neck pain often involves both the intervertebral disc and the facet joints simultaneously, based on a diagnostic combination of provocative discography and facet joint blocks.[9] However, provocative discography has more recently been reported to have an unacceptably high false-positive rate in patients with chronic pain,[10] potentially limiting the validity of these findings.

The C2-3 and C5-6 facet joints are the most commonly affected segments in cases of facet-mediated pain diagnosed by facet joint blocks.[8,11,12] However, the C2-3 and C5-6 joints have not been found to have the highest prevalence of facet arthrosis in cadaveric specimens. In 1 cadaveric study, facet arthrosis was found to increase with age, with the C4-5 level affected most frequently, followed by C3-4, C2-3, C5-6, and C6-7.[13] There is therefore a discrepancy between the joints clinically most affected and those that demonstrate the greatest prevalence of facet arthrosis.

ANATOMY

The zygapophyseal joints are 1 of 2 articulations between adjacent vertebrae; the other articulation is the intervertebral disc, which makes up a fibrocartilaginous joint or symphysis between adjacent vertebral bodies. The articular processes in the cervical spine are relatively bulky and form a column of bone that is separated by the zygapophyseal joints. Facets of the superior articular processes of 1 vertebra face the reciprocally oriented facets on the inferior articular facet of the vertebra above, forming the joint. The orientation of these facet joints influences the range of motion of the joint.

The intervertebral disc permits motion in all directions, and therefore the type of motion possible between a pair of adjacent vertebrae is determined by the zygapophyseal joints. The cervical zygapophyseal joints are ellipsoid, although the degrees of freedom of joint movement are influenced more by the orientation of the articular processes than the shape of the facets themselves. The articular facets on the superior and inferior processes slide relative to one another in flexion and extension of the spine, and also in lateral bending. Rotation is limited because of the more or less coronal orientation of the joints. This contrasts with the orientation of the zygapophyseal joints in the lumbar spine, in which the facet joints lie on a more sagittal plane.[14] The normal range of axial rotation in the entire cervical spine is approximately 70° to 90°, of which 40° to 45° are accomplished at the C1-C2 joint complex.[15] As true synovial joints, the facets are covered by articular cartilage and a thin capsule that is lined by a synovial membrane.

Between C3-4 and C7-T1, the zygapophyseal joint receives innervation from twigs of the posterior rami of spinal nerves associated with the 2 vertebral arches above and below. However, at C2-3, the joint is innervated by 2 different branches of the posterior ramus of C3—a medial branch termed the third occipital nerve—and a separate articular branch. The uppermost cervical synovial joints, the atlanto occipital joint and the atlanto axial joint, are innervated by branches of the C1 and C2 ventral rami rather than branches of the posterior rami.[16]

Histologic studies of human cadavers reveal the presence of abundant nerve fibers and nerve endings in the cervical facet joint capsule,[17] supporting its potential role in pain generation. A-delta and c fibers are clustered in the dorsolateral aspect of the facet joint capsule, near the attachment of tendons and muscles.[18] The presence of nerves reactive to substance P and calcitonin gene-related peptide, peptides important in the transmission and modulation of pain, lends additional support to the capsule as a potential pain generator. Mechanoreceptive nerve endings have been discovered in the capsule in addition to nociceptive nerve endings, suggesting that the capsule supplies input to the central nervous system regarding both proprioception and pain sensation.[19] Reflexes from these mechanoreceptors have been postulated to play an important role in the prevention of joint instability.[19] Interestingly, the presence of mechanoreceptors in the thoracic and lumbar spine is less consistent, suggesting the relative importance of the proprioceptive function of the cervical facet joints.[20] Further evaluation of the mechanoreceptors in the cervical spine reveals that they have a relatively large receptive field, such that 1 or 2 nerve endings may be sufficient to monitor the entire area of one individual facet capsule. Therefore, damage to even a small area may denervate a significant amount of the facet capsule, with potentially important long-term consequences. For instance, in a canine model of joint denervation, a deafferented limb led to accelerated development of arthropathy.[21] An average of 22.4% of the facet capsule is covered with muscle fibers, with slightly more muscular coverage in males than in females. Muscles insert directly onto the facet capsule, so direct loading of the facet capsule is possible with muscular contraction.[22]

CLINICAL PRESENTATION

The clinical presentation of pain arising from the facet joints is typically unilateral pain that does not radiate into the upper limb past the shoulder. Cervical rotation and extension may exacerbate the pain. The pattern of radiating pain was well described in a small number of asymptomatic volunteers by Dwyer and Bogduk[23] using noxious stimulation of the joints via injection of contrast medium into the joint itself, until pain was experienced. The injections produced a reasonably characteristic pattern of pain, which was subsequently validated in a series of patients with suspected facet-mediated pain who underwent diagnostic medial branch blocks.[24] Typical referral patterns are discussed in Chapter One, and are again shown in **Fig. 1**. As mentioned in earlier chapters, it is important to recognize the similar pattern of pain referral produced by noxious stimulation of both the cervical zygapophyseal joints and the cervical intervertebral discs.[25,26] As such, pain referral patterns cannot be used in isolation to determine whether neck pain is originating from the facet joint or another

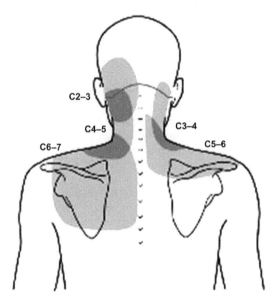

Fig. 1. The distribution of pain following stimulation of the zygapophyseal joints.

structure. However, the segmental level of pain can be reasonably assessed using the previously mentioned referral patterns. Pain arising from both the zygapophyseal joints and the intervertebral discs simultaneously should be considered.[9]

PHYSICAL EXAMINATION

Historically, evaluation of the patient with neck pain has included several physical examination components, including range-of-motion testing, palpation, segmental analysis, and a neurologic examination, as well as those mentioned in other articles of this issue. Indeed, a systematic review of patient expectations in the evaluation of spine pain reveals that patients expect a careful physical examination and are dissatisfied if this is not felt to be present.[27] However, several studies have shown poor interexaminer reliability of various components of the physical examination of the cervical spine.[28–34] A lone study in the setting of a chiropractic office[35] supports good interexaminer reliability for palpation of cervical facet joint. In 1998, Jull[36] reported 100% sensitivity and 100% specificity for diagnosing pain arising from the facet joints using manual diagnosis by a trained manipulative therapist. Diagnoses were confirmed by radiologically guided single diagnostic blocks. However, a larger, more recent follow-up study[37] using the same signs for segmental dysfunction as Jull but using controlled rather than single diagnostic blocks, found a lower level of validity. In this study, manual diagnosis resulted in high levels of sensitivity for pain arising from the C2-3 segment (sensitivity = 0.88) and C5-6 segment (sensitivity = 0.89), but a much lower specificity (specificity = 0.39 at C2-3, specificity = 0.50 at C5-6). Another recent study examining mechanical pressure pain thresholds found a low diagnostic accuracy in predicting symptomatic facet joints, using diagnostic medial branch blocks as a diagnostic gold standard. With very light pressure of 1 kPa, the diagnostic accuracy was 38%, which increased to an accuracy of 67% when using moderate pressure of 30 kPa.[38]

When manual examination is undertaken, palpation of the posterior elements is most easily accomplished with the patient supine. The spinous processes of C2, C6, and C7 are the most obvious bony landmarks. Palpating the occiput and descending in the midline, the first protuberance encountered is the spinous process of C2. While the spinous processes of C3, C4, and C5 may be appreciated with careful technique and flexion of the spine, the spinous processes of C6 and C7 are the next obvious structures appreciated in the midline. The spinous processes of C6 and C7 may be distinguished by passive flexion and extension of the neck; the C6 spinous process tends to be more mobile in relation to the relatively fixed C7 spinous process. The facet joints may be palpated approximately 1.3 to 2.5 cm lateral to the spinous process, and are not felt as discrete structures but rather hard bony masses under the fingers.[15]

Physical examination of the cervical spine, therefore, has not been shown to be effective in accurately diagnosing pain arising from the zygapophyseal joints. Nonetheless, a complete physical examination and neurologic evaluation should be performed to assess for the presence of radiculopathy, spinal cord injury, brachial plexus injury, vascular pathology, shoulder injury, or traumatic brain injury, especially in the setting of trauma; several tests with good specificity and sensitivity accurately predict the presence of a cervical radiculopathy.[39]

DIFFERENTIAL DIAGNOSIS

As the typical presentation of facet-mediated pain is unilateral neck pain without radiation into the upper limb past the shoulder, a differential diagnosis should focus on neck pain syndromes rather than etiologies involving symptoms radiating into the arm such as radiculopathy and myelopathy. Review of the differential diagnosis of neck pain is covered in other articles in this issue.

DIAGNOSTIC INJECTIONS

The current gold standard for diagnosis of facet-mediated pain uses blinded, controlled diagnostic medial branch blocks. A working diagnosis of facet-mediated pain can theoretically be confirmed by injection of local anesthetic around the medial branches of the dorsal primary rami that supply the joint. However, there is no consensus about what constitutes a positive diagnostic block. Comparative blocks using anesthetics with different durations (eg, lidocaine and bupivacaine) have been advocated by some authors based on high false-positive rates (27% to 63%) using single diagnostic blocks alone.[40] Using comparative blocks, a positive diagnosis is made only if there is concordant response to the different anesthetics (ie, a longer duration of pain relief with the longer-acting anesthetic). While there are clear theoretical advantages to this approach, other authors do not support the double-block paradigm, arguing that a single positive diagnostic block is adequate, and that the use of 2 separate injections represents additional risk and cost to the patient.[41,42] Regardless of whether single or comparative blocks are employed, these diagnostic blocks are frequently performed before therapeutic radiofrequency denervation or other interventional treatments.

IMAGING OF THE ZYGAPOPHYSEAL JOINTS

Facet joint abnormalities can be demonstrated on various common imaging modalities, including plain films, computed tomography (CT), and magnetic resonance imaging (MRI). As noted previously, however, population-based studies of patients with neck pain who underwent radiographs of the cervical spine failed to show a relationship between facet osteoarthritis and neck pain in men or women between the ages of 20 and 65.[43] CT imaging has a higher degree of accuracy in determination of the precise degree of facet arthrosis.[44] However this determination has a limited degree of clinical utility in the diagnosis of pain or the prediction of response to treatment. Findings on CT imaging are unable to predict responses to facet joint blocks.[45] Similarly, MRI findings are unable to predict response to treatment with radiofrequency denervation in patients with facet joint pain diagnosed by medial branch blocks.[41]

Bone scintigraphy using single photon emission CT (SPECT) has been more recently advocated as having the ability to identify patients who will respond favorably to facet joint injections. A study using SPECT scans of the lumbar spine found that 87% of patients with a positive SPECT scan who underwent facet joint injection met clinical criteria for improvement at 1 month after intervention, versus only 13% of those patients with a negative SPECT scan who underwent facet joint injection.[46] These findings have not been replicated in the cervical spine.

WHIPLASH

The term whiplash dates to 1928, when it was used at a conference by the American orthopedic surgeon Harold Crowe[47] to describe the effects of an acceleration–deceleration mechanism, including a lash-like effect in the neck. While Crowe himself denounced the term 34 years later,[48] because he perceived its misapplication among physicians, patients, and attorneys, it continues to be widely used both within the medical community and in public discourse. The term whiplash may be defined as an acceleration–deceleration mechanism of energy transfer to the neck that results from rear-end or side-impact motor vehicle collisions. Subsequent bone and soft tissue injuries related to this have been termed whiplash-associated disorder (WAD), and although various symptoms have been suggested as components of chronic WAD, including cognitive disturbances, visual changes, and dizziness, the chief constituents remain cervical pain and headaches.

Whiplash injuries constitute the most common disorders associated with motor vehicle accidents (MVAs) in US emergency departments, making up more than 25% of all injuries to motor vehicle occupants treated in the emergency department in 2000.[49] The chronicity of patient complaints related to WAD varies widely. One report from Lithuania found that only 8% of patients involved in a rear impact MVA had chronic neck or headache pain 1 to 3 years after the accident, which was not significantly different than a group of controls.[50] Other studies have found rates of chronic neck pain as high as 52% at 1 year following MVA.[51] The most recent systematic review to report on prognostic factors for development of chronic pain following whiplash found moderate evidence for association with high initial pain intensity, pain-related disability, and cold hyperalgesia.[52] Inconclusive association exists for decreased neck range of motion and radicular symptoms. Factors that do not appear to influence outcome include age, female gender, rear-end collision, and compensation.[53]

In patients who present with chronic neck pain following whiplash injuries, the facet joints appear to be the most common source of pain; the prevalence of facet-mediated pain in this population is 54%, based on comparative facet joint blocks.[11] Fractures of the articular pillars, which may not be visible on standard radiographs, have been reported after MVAs, as have tears of the joint capsule and hemarthrosis of the facet joints.[54] Headaches, a common component of WAD, are often due to referred pain from the C2-3 facet joint in this setting. Comparative blocks identified the C2-3 joint as responsible for whiplash-associated headache pain in 50% of cases.[8] The basis for chronic neck pain following a whiplash injury not related to the facet joints includes a number of potential structures, including the intervertebral discs, spinal ligaments, spinal ganglia, and cervical muscles, as well as psychosocial factors.

WHIPLASH BIOMECHANICS

Indirect evidence of the importance of forces transmitted through the neck in the development of whiplash syndrome comes from analysis of antiwhiplash seats designed to reduce these forces. Active head restraints move upwards and closer to the driver's head during a rear impact, to provide earlier head and neck support. These headrests have resulted in significant reductions in whiplash claims, with reductions between 43% and 75%.[55,56]

The complex biomechanical forces occurring during whiplash injuries are well described in both in cadaveric and animal models. The facet joints undergo shear forces, compression, tension, flexion, and extension at different levels of the neck and at different times during the event.[57] Following a rear impact, the cervical spine attains a nonphysiologic S-shape configuration, with the occiput to C2 initially in flexion as the head lags behind the extending cervical spine, maintaining its static inertia. This occurs at approximately 60 milliseconds after the impact. In later stages, at approximately 100 milliseconds after impact, the entire cervical spine is in an extension mode.[58] The lower cervical facet joints respond to these forces by undergoing both shear and distraction anteriorly, with the posterior aspect of the joints undergoing shear and compression.[59] Following extension, the head is accelerated forward, forcing the entire neck into flexion. As the velocity of the impact increases, the forces generated at impact are similarly increased. With an impact velocity of 5 mph, peak horizontal acceleration forces of 4 to 5 G (4 to 5 times the acceleration due to the force of gravity) are experienced,[60] similar to the amount of acceleration experienced at the bottom of a roller-coaster loop. With an impact velocity of 20 mph, the head reaches a peak acceleration of 12 G. Positioning the head in a flexed or rotated position during impact significantly increases the measured facet capsular strains. Capsule strains in these positions are roughly double those with the neck in neutral, a finding potentially consistent with greater symptom severity and duration observed in whiplash patients who have their head turned at impact.[61]

The two main postulated mechanisms for facet joint injury during whiplash are synovial fold impingement and capsular strain.

Synovial folds are well innervated with nociceptive fibers,[62] supporting their potential role in pain production. This theory postulates that the synovial fold is pinched between the subchondral bone of the superior and inferior facet processes during the nonphysiologic movement of the cervical facets. The instantaneous axis of rotation of the vertebral bodies in a simulated whiplash setting is shifted superiorly, which increases posterior compressive forces. With an upwardly shifted axis of rotation, the posterior edge of the inferior facet on the more cephalad vertebra collides with the superior articular facet of the vertebra below it.[63] In another experimental model, the posterior region of the joint was found to compress more than the anterior region, and the varying kinematics at the 2 ends of the joint resulted in a pinching mechanism.[64]

The theory of capsular strain, an alternative mechanism for pain production in whiplash injuries, has received more attention than synovial fold impingement. Capsular strain has been found to increase with shear loading such as that experienced in

MVAs,[65] and partial rupture has occurred at 35% to 65% of maximal capsular strain.[66] As noted previously, muscular attachments cover an average of 22.4% of the surface of the facet joint capsule, and direct contraction will therefore load the joint. Loading due to muscular contraction has been estimated at 27 N for males and 15 N for females. With a scaling factor of 1.5 to account for rapid muscle elongation such as may occur during whiplash, capsular loading forces have been calculated to be approximately 51 N in males and 36 N in females. The capsular force generated passively by simulated whiplash events is approximately 14 N. Summing these forces, the total calculated joint forces of approximately 65 N in males and 50 N in females fall within the range of forces associated with partial rupture of the facet capsule, which has been documented to occur between 48 N and 121 N.[22]

In an animal model of capsular damage, subfailure capsular injury in rats produced sustained hyperalgesia, whereas complete capsular failure produced only a transient pain response.[67] These data suggest that sensory input from an intact capsule is important in the maintenance of a pain signal. Following this model, a more intense mechanical stress may not produce a worse pain syndrome; lower stresses may counterintuitively produce longer-lasting pain. Studies corroborating these findings in humans have yet to be performed. However, they lend further theoretical support to the treatment of chronic facet-mediated pain by elimination of the sensory input from the joints with radiofrequency ablation.

Indeed, there is now good evidence to support radiofrequency ablation in relieving pain in patients with chronic whiplash-associated neck pain. A randomized, double-blind trial in patients with chronic whiplash-associated neck pain compared active radiofrequency ablation with a sham procedure, where the probe was placed in position but not turned on. The median time that elapsed before the pain returned to 50% of the preoperative level was 263 days in the active-treatment group and 8 days in the control group. At 27 weeks, 58% of patients in the active-treatment group and 8% of patients in the control group were pain free.[68]

SUMMARY

The importance of the cervical zygapophyseal joints in the evaluation of neck pain is clear. In chronic neck pain, the facet joints are responsible for 25% to 65% of pain complaints, and 50% to 60% of complaints in chronic, traumatically induced pain. The C2-3 and C5-6 joints are most frequently affected, and relatively consistent pain referral distributions can assist in identification of the painful level. Physical examination of the facet joints, while expected and valued by patients, has not been shown to be reliable in detection of facet pathology. Plain films, CT, scans, and MRI studies, while able to clearly define anatomic changes, do not correlate with painful joints or response to treatment. More research remains to be done in defining the role of SPECT scans in predicting whether cervical facet joints will be responsive to treatment; currently the gold standard for diagnosis of facet-mediated pain remains diagnostic anesthetic injections. An understanding of the biomechanics of whiplash-associated neck pain, as presented here, continues to evolve, although prediction of patients who will develop chronic symptoms remains unreliable based on history, examination, psychosocial, and imaging findings.

REFERENCES

1. Orr WS, Young JR, Jardine A, et al. Orr's circle of the sciences: a series of treatsies on the principles of science, with their application to practical pursuits. London: W.S. Orr and Company; 1854.

2. Oxford English Dictionary. Oxford University Press; 2011 [Online]. Available at: http://www.oed.com.offcampus.lib.washington.edu/view/Entry/233132?redirectedFrom= zygapophysis. Accessed March 27, 2011.

3. Haldeman S, Carroll LJ, Cassidy JD. The empowerment of people with neck pain: introduction. The bone and joint decade 2000–2010 task force on neck pain and its associated disorders. J Manipulative Physiol Ther 2009;32(Suppl 2):S10–6.

4. Hogg-Johnson S, van der Velde G, Carroll LJ, et al. The burden and determinants of neck pain in the general population: results of the bone and joint decade 2000–2010 task force on neck pain and its associated disorders. J Manipulative Physiol Ther 2009;32(Suppl 2):S46–60.

5. Côté P, van der Velde G, Cassidy JD, et al. The burden and determinants of neck pain in workers: results of the bone and joint decade 2000–2010 task force on neck pain and its associated disorders. Spine (Phila Pa 1976) 2008;33(Suppl 4):S60–74.

6. Janwantanakul P, Pensri P, Jiamjarasrangsri V, et al. Prevalence of self-reported musculoskeletal symptoms among office workers. Occup Med (Lond) 2008; 58(6):436–8.

7. Kirpalani D, Mitra R. Cervical facet joint dysfunction: a review. Arch Phys Med Rehabil 2008;89(4):770–4.

8. Lord SM, Barnsley L, Wallis BJ, et al. Chronic cervical zygapophysial joint pain after whiplash. A placebo-controlled prevalence study. Spine (Phila Pa 1976) 1996;21(15):1737–44 [discussion: 1744–5].

9. Bogduk N, Aprill C. On the nature of neck pain, discography and cervical zygapophysial joint blocks. Pain 1993;54(2):213–7.

10. Carragee EJ, Tanner CM, Khurana S, et al. The rates of false-positive lumbar discography in select patients without low back symptoms. Spine (Phila Pa 1976) 2000;25(11):1373–80 [discussion: 1381].

11. Barnsley L, Lord SM, Wallis BJ, et al. The prevalence of chronic cervical zygapophysial joint pain after whiplash. Spine (Phila Pa 1976) 1995;20(1):20–5 [discussion: 26].

12. Bogduk N, Lord SM. Cervical spine disorders. Curr Opin Rheumatol 1998;10(2): 110–5.

13. Lee MJ, Riew KD. The prevalence cervical facet arthrosis: an osseous study in a cadveric population. Spine J 2009;9(9):711–4.

14. Rosse C, Gaddum-Rosse P, Hollinshead WH. Hollinshead's textbook of anatomy. Philadelphia: Lippincott-Raven Publishers; 1997.

15. Magee DJ. Orthopedic physical assessment. Philadelphia: Saunders; 2002.

16. Bogduk N. The clinical anatomy of the cervical dorsal rami. Spine (Phila Pa 1976) 1982;7(4):319–30.

17. Kallakuri S, Singh A, Chen C, et al. Demonstration of substance P, calcitonin gene-related peptide, and protein gene product 9.5 containing nerve fibers in human cervical facet joint capsules. Spine (Phila Pa 1976) 2004;29(11):1182–6.

18. Chen C, Lu Y, Kallakuri S, et al. Distribution of A-delta and C-fiber receptors in the cervical facet joint capsule and their response to stretch. J Bone Joint Surg Am 2006;88(8):1807–16.

19. McLain RF. Mechanoreceptor endings in human cervical facet joints. Spine (Phila Pa 1976) 1994;19(5):495–501.

20. McLain RF, Pickar JG. Mechanoreceptor endings in human thoracic and lumbar facet joints. Spine (Phila Pa 1976) 1998;23(2):168–73.

21. O'Connor BL, Palmoski MJ, Brandt KD. Neurogenic acceleration of degenerative joint lesions. J Bone Joint Surg Am 1985;67(4):562–72.

22. Winkelstein BA, McLendon RE, Barbir A, et al. An anatomical investigation of the human cervical facet capsule, quantifying muscle insertion area. J Anat 2001; 198:455–61.

23. Dwyer A, Aprill C, Bogduk N. Cervical zygapophyseal joint pain patterns. I: a study in normal volunteers. Spine (Phila Pa 1976) 1990;15(6):453–7.

24. Aprill C, Dwyer A, Bogduk N. Cervical zygapophyseal joint pain patterns. II: a clinical evaluation. Spine (Phila Pa 1976) 1990;15(6):458–61.

25. Grubb SA, Kelly CK. Cervical discography: clinical implications from 12 years of experience. Spine (Phila Pa 1976) 2000;25(11):1382–9.

26. Schellhas KP, Smith MD, Gundry CR, et al. Cervical discogenic pain. Prospective correlation of magnetic resonance imaging and discography in asymptomatic subjects and pain sufferers. Spine (Phila Pa 1976) 1996;21(3):300–11 [discussion: 311–2].

27. Verbeek J, Sengers MJ, Riemens L, et al. Patient expectations of treatment for back pain: a systematic review of qualitative and quantitative studies. Spine (Phila Pa 1976) 2004;29(20):2309–18.

28. Deboer KF, Harmon R Jr, Tuttle CD, et al. Reliability study of detection of somatic dysfunctions in the cervical spine. J Manipulative Physiol Ther 1985;8(1):9–16.

29. Fjellner A, Bexander C, Faleij R, et al. Interexaminer reliability in physical examination of the cervical spine. J Manipulative Physiol Ther 1999;22(8):511–6.

30. Malanga GA, Landes P, Nadler SF. Provocative tests in cervical spine examination: historical basis and scientific analyses. Pain Physician 2003;6(2): 199–205.

31. Nansel DD, Peneff AL, Jansen RD, et al. Interexaminer concordance in detecting joint-play asymmetries in the cervical spines of otherwise asymptomatic subjects. J Manipulative Physiol Ther 1989;12(6):428–33.

32. Pool JJ, Hoving JL, de Vet HC, et al. The interexaminer reproducibility of physical examination of the cervical spine. J Manipulative Physiol Ther 2004;27(2): 84–90.

33. Strender LE, Lundin M, Nell K. Interexaminer reliability in physical examination of the neck. J Manipulative Physiol Ther 1997;20(8):516–20.

34. Youdas JW, Carey JR, Garrett TR. Reliability of measurements of cervical spine range of motion–comparison of three methods. Phys Ther 1991;71(2):98–104 [discussion: 105–6].

35. Hubka MJ, Phelan SP. Interexaminer reliability of palpation for cervical spine tenderness. J Manipulative Physiol Ther 1994;17(9):591–5.

36. Jull G, Bogduk N, Marsland A. The accuracy of manual diagnosis for cervical zygapophysial joint pain syndromes. Med J Aust 1988;148(5):233–6.

37. King W, Lau P, Lees R, et al. The validity of manual examination in assessing patients with neck pain. Spine J 2007;7(1):22–6.

38. Siegenthaler A, Eichenberger U, Schmidlin K, et al. What does local tenderness say about the origin of pain? An investigation of cervical zygapophysial joint pain. Anesth Analg 2010;110(3):923–7.

39. Wainner RS, Fritz JM, Irrgang JJ, et al. Reliability and diagnostic accuracy of the clinical examination and patient self-report measures for cervical radiculopathy. Spine (Phila Pa 1976) 2003;28(1):52–62.

40. Falco FJ, Erhart S, Wargo BW, et al. Systematic review of diagnostic utility and therapeutic effectiveness of cervical facet joint interventions. Pain Physician 2009;12(2):323–44.

41. Cohen SP, Bajwa ZH, Kraemer JJ, et al. Factors predicting success and failure for cervical facet radiofrequency denervation: a multi-center analysis. Reg Anesth Pain Med 2007;32(6):495–503.

42. van Eerd M, Patijn J, Lataster A, et al. Cervical facet pain. Pain Pract 2010;10(2): 113–23.
43. van der Donk J, Schouten JS, Passchier J, et al. The associations of neck pain with radiological abnormalities of the cervical spine and personality traits in a general population. J Rheumatol 1991;18(12):1884–9.
44. Lehman RA Jr, Helgeson MD, Keeler KA, et al. Comparison of magnetic resonance imaging and computed tomography in predicting facet arthrosis in the cervical spine. Spine (Phila Pa 1976) 2009;34(1):65–8.
45. Hechelhammer L, Pfirrmann CW, Zanetti M, et al. Imaging findings predicting the outcome of cervical facet joint blocks. Eur Radiol 2007;17(4):959–64.
46. Pneumaticos SG, Chatziioannou SN, Hipp JA, et al. Low back pain: prediction of short-term outcome of facet joint injection with bone scintigraphy. Radiology 2006;238(2):693–8.
47. Evans RW. Whiplash around the world. Headache 1995;35(5):262–3.
48. Crowe H. A new diagnostic sign in neck injuries. Calif Med 1964;100:12–3.
49. Quinlan KP, Annest JL, Myers B, et al. Neck strains and sprains among motor vehicle occupants-United States, 2000. Accid Anal Prev 2004;36(1):21–7.
50. Schrader H, Obelieniene D, Bovim G, et al. Natural evolution of late whiplash syndrome outside the medicolegal context. Lancet 1996;347(9010): 1207–11.
51. Pobereskin LH. Whiplash following rear end collisions: a prospective cohort study. J Neurol Neurosurg Psychiatr 2005;76(8):1146–51.
52. Williams M, Williamson E, Gates S, et al. A systematic literature review of physical prognostic factors for the development of late whiplash syndrome. Spine (Phila Pa 1976) 2007;32(25):E764–80.
53. Scholten-Peeters GG, Verhagen AP, Bekkering GE, et al. Prognostic factors of whiplash-associated disorders: a systematic review of prospective cohort studies. Pain 2003;104:303–22.
54. Barnsley L, Lord S, Bogduk N. Whiplash injury. Pain 1994;58(3):283–307.
55. Farmer CM, Wells JK, Lund AK. Effects of head restraint and seat redesign on neck injury risk in rear-end crashes. Traffic Inj Prev 2003;4(2):83–90.
56. Viano DC, Olsen S. The effectiveness of active head restraint in preventing whiplash. J Trauma 2001;51(5):959–69.
57. Tencer AF, Mirza S, Bensel K. Internal loads in the cervical spine during motor vehicle rear-end impacts: the effect of acceleration and head-to-head restraint proximity. Spine (Phila Pa 1976) 2002;27(1):34–42.
58. Cusick JF, Pintar FA, Yoganandan N. Whiplash syndrome: kinematic factors influencing pain patterns. Spine (Phila Pa 1976) 2001;26(11):1252–8.
59. Stemper BD, Yoganandan N, Pintar FA. Gender- and region-dependent local facet joint kinematics in rear impact: implications in whiplash injury. Spine (Phila Pa 1976) 2004;29(16):1764–71.
60. Allen ME, Weir-Jones I, Motiuk DR, et al. Acceleration perturbations of daily living. A comparison to whiplash. Spine (Phila Pa 1976) 1994;19(11):1285–90.
61. Siegmund GP, Davis MB, Quinn KP, et al. Head-turned postures increase the risk of cervical facet capsule injury during whiplash. Spine (Phila Pa 1976) 2008; 33(15):1643–9.
62. Inami S, Shiga T, Tsujino A, et al. Immunohistochemical demonstration of nerve fibers in the synovial fold of the human cervical facet joint. J Orthop Res 2001; 19(4):593–6.
63. Kaneoka K, Ono K, Inami S, et al. Motion analysis of cervical vertebrae during whiplash loading. Spine (Phila Pa 1976) 1999;24(8):763–9 [discussion: 770].

64. Yoganandan N, Pintar FA, Cusick JF. Biomechanical analyses of whiplash injuries using an experimental model. Accid Anal Prev 2002;34(5):663–71.
65. Siegmund GP, Myers BS, Davis MB, et al. Mechanical evidence of cervical facet capsule injury during whiplash: a cadaveric study using combined shear, compression, and extension loading. Spine (Phila Pa 1976) 2001;26(19): 2095–101.
66. Winkelstein BA, Nightingale RW, Richardson WJ, et al. The cervical facet capsule and its role in whiplash injury: a biomechanical investigation. Spine (Phila Pa 1976) 2000;25(10):1238–46.
67. Lee KE, Franklin AN, Davis MB, et al. Tensile cervical facet capsule ligament mechanics: failure and subfailure responses in the rat. J Biomech 2006;39(7): 1256–64.
68. Lord SM, Barnsley L, Wallis BJ, et al. Percutaneous radio-frequency neurotomy for chronic cervical zygapophyseal-joint pain. N Engl J Med 1996;335(23): 1721–6.

Cervical Spine Pain in the Competitive Athlete

Brian J. Krabak, MD, MBA[a],*, Samantha L. Kanarek, DO, MS[b]

KEYWORDS

• Cervical • Spine • Athlete

Cervical pain is a common complaint in both the well-conditioned athlete and the weekend warrior. Some injuries are mild in nature, responding to conservative treatment, including rest, medication, physical therapy, and time. However, more serious injuries, especially those involving the cervical spine, can have devastating consequences. Having a comprehensive understanding of the evaluation and management of cervical pain and cervical spine emergencies is crucial for physicians providing coverage for organized athletic events or for those who serve as team physicians. This article reviews the common causes of cervical spine pain in the competitive athlete.

CERVICAL SPINE EMERGENCIES

Over the past few decades, the increase in size, weight, and agility of athletes combined with advances in equipment technology has led to a potential increase in the risk of severe cervical spine injuries.[1,2] Football, ice hockey, wrestling, diving, skiing, snowboarding, cheerleading, and rugby represent some of the sporting activities with the largest risk of catastrophic cervical spine injuries.[3] The most common mechanisms of severe cervical spine injury during these athletic events involve flexion or extension of the cervical spine with axial loading. Flexion with axial loading results in loss of cervical spine lordosis, leading to transmission of extreme axial forces after an impact to the top of the head that can result in severe spinal and neurologic injury.[4] One example includes spear tackling in football, when the athlete uses the dome of the head as an initial point of contact, thus placing the cervical spine in flexion with

Financial disclosure: There are no financial disclosures for either author.
[a] Rehabilitation, Orthopaedics and Sports Medicine, University of Washington and Seattle Children's Sports Medicine, Seattle, WA, USA
[b] Rehabilitation Medicine, University of Washington, 1959 NE Pacific Street, Box 356490, Seattle, WA 98195, USA
* Corresponding author. University of Washington Sports and Spine Physicians, 4245 NE Roosevelt Way, Box 354740, Seattle, WA 98105.
E-mail address: bkrabak@uw.edu

axial loading. Athletes who spear tackle repeatedly become prone to the development of spear tackler's spine, involving reversal of the normal cervical spine lordosis, stenosis of the cervical spinal canal, and posttraumatic bony changes. These changes can increase the risk of sustaining permanent neurologic injury following axial loading.[5]

In 1975, the National Football Head and Neck Injury Registry was created for the purpose of tracking the extent of severe head and neck injuries.[4] Soon thereafter, Torg and colleagues[6] retrospectively gathered data on the incidence of such injuries and found an increasing number of catastrophic cervical spine injuries between 1975 and 1978. These findings were attributed to improved design and protective capabilities of helmets. The incidence of head injuries decreased after the helmet modifications. However, athletes began spear tackling with increased frequency, placing the cervical spine and spinal cord at a higher risk of injury. The data collected revealed that 52% of the cervical spine injuries with resultant tetraplegia were the direct result of spear tackling or a direct force applied to the helmet (from blocking or tackling).[6] After interpretation of these findings, the National Collegiate Athletic Association and the National Federation of State High School Associations implemented rule changes in 1976 that prohibited using the helmet as the initial point of contact for blocking or tackling.[4] The incidence of catastrophic cervical spine injuries with associated tetraplegia has decreased significantly since the implementation of these rules. There were a total of 32 and 34 catastrophic injuries in 1975 and 1976, respectively. The number of catastrophic injuries decreased to 12 in 1977. Overall, the number of catastrophic injuries remains low, with 10 such injuries in 2006 and 8 in 2007.[7]

Despite the low numbers of catastrophic cervical injuries over the past few decades, the team physician still needs to be prepared for a possible spinal cord injury. It is imperative that the sports physician pays attention to the field of play to optimize the possibility of witnessing the mechanism of injury. These injuries can be quite dramatic, requiring the medical staff to respond quickly and efficiently to minimize the extent of the injury. A well-coordinated emergency plan should be implemented before the start of an athletic season and rehearsed so that each member of the team understands his or her role. The emergency plan discussion should include physicians, trainers, emergency medical staff, and coaches. Key points include emergency equipment location, process for stabilizing the athlete, evacuation route, and location of the nearest medical facility.

In a patient suspected of having a severe cervical spine injury, a stepwise approach is necessary to assure proper care. The initial evaluation should consist of assessing hemodynamic stability (airway, breathing, circulation [ABC]) followed by a complete assessment of neurologic status. The neck must be immobilized until cervical spine injury is ruled out, and unconscious athletes should be assumed to have a cervical spine injury until proven otherwise. Secondary survey is performed once the athlete arrives at the emergency department.[4]

During the on-field evaluation, the physician should take into consideration any equipment that may be affecting spine stabilization. In football and hockey players, helmet and shoulder pads should initially remain in place while maintaining immobilization of the cervical spine. Removal of the helmet with the shoulder pads in place results in relative extension of the cervical spine. Removal of the shoulder pads with the helmet in place results in relative flexion of the cervical spine. Thus, keeping the helmet and shoulder pads in place allows the cervical spine to maintain a more neutral position.[8] Further removal of protective equipment should occur in a monitored setting by a physician with proper experience. If needed for airway management, the face mask or shield can be removed during the on-field assessment via a cordless screwdriver or quick release. The airway should be cleared with a jaw thrust maneuver, avoiding head tilt. Toler and colleagues[9] found that insertion of a pocket mask between the player's chin and face mask provides an adequate seal for performing modified jaw thrust and rescue breathing through the bars of the face mask.

In the conscious athlete, the secondary assessment should include a history taking and physical examination on the field to evaluate for upper and lower extremity pain (bilateral or unilateral), cervical pain, weakness, numbness, and paresthesias.[4] Gentle cervical active range of motion should be considered, but passive range of motion should be avoided unless it is clear that there is no significant injury. Concerning signs or symptoms include focal neurologic findings, severe cervical spine tenderness or pain, rigid cervical spasm, and persistent apprehension. These findings suggest that cervical injury and management should proceed with maintaining spine immobilization, continued ABC monitoring, and transportation to the local emergency department. As previously noted, helmet and shoulder pads should be removed by appropriately trained professionals only when the patient is in a controlled environment.

Once the athlete has been transported to the emergency department, a complete neurologic examination, including the American Spinal Injury Association classification, as appropriate, should be repeated. Imaging, including cervical spine radiographs (anteroposterior, lateral, and odontoid), should be obtained. If the C7-T1 level is unable to be visualized (shoulder pads often interfere with visualization of the inferior cervical spine) or there is a concern for fracture on radiographs, a computed tomographic (CT) scan of the cervical spine should be obtained. Magnetic resonance imaging (MRI) of the cervical spine is warranted in those with suggested cervical spinal cord injury.[4] Immobilization of the spine should begin on the playing field, continue through transport and evaluation in the emergency department, and terminate only after a cervical spine injury is either ruled out with the appropriate imaging or definitively stabilized.[10]

There are circumstances in which a cervical spine injury can be cleared without obtaining radiographs. The National Emergency X-Ray Use Study (NEXUS) found that a patient with no midline cervical spine tenderness, no focal neurologic deficits, no distracting injuries, normal alertness, and no intoxication had a low probability of cervical spine injury. Patients with the earlier-mentioned criteria who are fully conscious can be cleared without radiographs.[11] In a prospective Canadian study, patients were found to have a low risk of cervical spinal injury if they had no limitation of cervical rotation (45° in either direction), met a list of 3 criteria (younger than 65 years, no dangerous mechanism of injury, and no upper extremity paresthesias), and had 1 of the following: a simple rear-end motor vehicle collision, the ability to tolerate a sitting position in the emergency department, the ability to ambulate at any time, delayed onset of cervical pain, or absence of midline neck tenderness.[12] Although the Canadian study was found to have superior sensitivity and specificity than the NEXUS study,[13] both were designed for trauma patients who were being evaluated in the emergency department rather than for athletes on the playing field. Although it is possible to clear an athlete from a serious cervical spine injury using the earlier-mentioned criteria, it may not indicate a safe return to play. Athletes who are deemed to have minor cervical injuries should have full painless range of motion and full upper extremity strength before consideration for return to competition.

On-the-field evaluation of cervical spine injury should include an initial assessment of ABC, level of consciousness, and apprehension. Athletes with midline cervical tenderness, neurologic deficits, severe cervical pain, or rigidity should be immobilized and transported to a nearby emergency department for further neurologic and radiological evaluation and management.

STINGERS

Stingers, also known as "burners," are brachial plexus injuries caused by traction on the brachial plexus or compression of the cervical nerve roots. These injuries commonly occur in football. Lateral flexion of the neck with depression of the contralateral shoulder results in traction to the brachial plexus. The upper trunk is the most common area of the brachial plexus that is injured during a stinger injury. Extreme lateral flexion of the neck on the ipsilateral side narrows the neural foramen and can result in compression of the cervical nerve root.[14] The most common cervical nerve roots involved are C5 and C6 because they are the shortest (C5 is shorter than C6) and are in direct alignment with the upper trunk of the brachial plexus.[15] Stingers can result in transient neuropraxia, which can manifest with burning pain radiating down the arm and weakness of muscles innervated by the upper cervical nerve roots or the upper trunk of the brachial plexus. Commonly affected muscles are the deltoid, supraspinatus, infraspinatus, biceps brachii, brachioradialis, pronator teres, and wrist extensors.[16] The injured athlete is typically visualized shaking the involved extremity, with it hanging limply while leaning toward the side of injury.

Stingers are often self-limiting injuries that do not require intervention beyond keeping the athlete out of competition until neurologic signs and symptoms have resolved. Some athletes may have residual upper extremity weakness for up to several weeks, even after resolution of sensory symptoms. Although athletes who have sustained stingers are at an increased risk of sustaining additional stingers, they are not at an increased risk of sustaining serious cervical spine injury.[17] Neck rolls, also known as cowboy collars, are often used by football players who have sustained multiple stingers. The cowboy collars should be fitted properly to avoid excessive cervical motion. The efficacy of these collars in preventing stingers is controversial. Gorden and colleagues[18] showed that although the cowboy collar provided the greatest reduction in hyperextension of all football collars in production, none of them reduced lateral flexion. The efficacy of football collars in preventing stingers has not been studied.

Athletes who have sustained a stinger may return to competition after return of full strength in the affected extremity and resolution of neurologic symptoms. This usually takes several minutes but may require weeks. Patients who have persistent neurologic symptoms, involvement of bilateral upper extremities, persistent neck pain, or limited cervical spine range of motion should be assumed to have a cervical spine injury until proven otherwise.[19]

Further testing should be considered in athletes with persisting symptoms, continuing neurologic deficits, or repeated stingers. Cervical spine radiographs should include flexion and extension and anteroposterior and lateral views to rule out bony neuroforaminal stenosis or instability. For those in whom cervical nerve root injury is suspected, cervical MRI can be obtained to better identify neuroforaminal narrowing or the presence of a herniated disk. CT myelography can be helpful for identifying nerve root or neuroforaminal involvement. In cases with suspected recurrent or significant brachial plexus injury, MRI of the brachial plexus may be useful for identifying focal plexus pathology or ruling out a mass lesion.[20] Young athletes with persisting symptoms associated with a herniated disk should be advised to not return to contact sports until symptoms have resolved and appropriate rehabilitation has been completed.[20] Some of these athletes with significant neuroforaminal stenosis or cervical spine instability, despite complete resolution of symptoms and neurologic deficits, may be advised to refrain from returning to contact sports permanently.[20]

Although most athletes with stingers do not require electrodiagnostic testing for assessment, it can be helpful for the athlete with persisting weakness. Deltoid weakness is a very common clinical finding in this group of athletes. In athletes with marked muscle weakness presenting at 72 hours after injury, electrodiagnostic studies can demonstrate abnormalities indicating axon loss.[15] However, the optimal time frame for performing a study is 2 to 4 weeks after injury because electrodiagnostic findings of denervation may not present until 2 weeks after injury and can take 4 to 5 weeks to maximize.[15] Electrodiagnosis can help differentiate between a C5 or C6 radiculopathy and an upper trunk brachial plexopathy because these conditions are often very difficult to distinguish from each other based on clinical evaluation alone.[15] Further discussion about electrodiagnosis of neck and arm pain is covered in another article by Plastaras and colleagues elsewhere in this issue. Prolonged weakness may occur after a stinger injury without electromyographic (EMG) evidence of significant axon loss, suggesting a neuropraxia, which is associated with a more favorable prognosis.[20] On the other hand, EMG evidence of axon loss can be found in muscles with full clinical strength. These EMG abnormalities can persist for up to more than 4 years after the injury and after complete clinical recovery. These abnormalities are thus not helpful for determining safe return to play.[15] As such, clinical examination and evaluation for structural defects that may increase the risk of neurologic injury remain the methods of choice for making return-to-participation decisions.

CERVICAL CORD NEUROPRAXIA

Cervical cord neuropraxia is a transient neurologic event in which neurologic symptoms involve bilateral upper extremities, bilateral lower extremities, all 4 extremities, or the ipsilateral upper and lower extremities. Both sensory and motor nerves can be involved, and paresthesias, paresis, and neuropathic pain are common symptoms.[17] Neuropraxia is often referred to as a spinal cord concussion caused by the transient nature of the symptoms. Transient quadriparesis is the term used for neuropraxia involving all 4 extremities and has been found to occur in football, wrestling, basketball, boxing, and hockey. The time frame for resolution of symptoms can range from 10 minutes to 48 hours.[21]

Several mechanisms of injury have been suggested as a cause of cervical cord neuropraxia. Axial loading of the cervical spine while in flexion or hyperextension is the most commonly suggested mechanism of injury. It is thought that the movement of one vertebra on top of another during this extreme flexion or extension causes narrowing of the spinal canal, resulting in a "pincher" mechanism.[17] Infolding of the ligamentum flavum can occur during hyperextension and has been shown to decrease the spinal canal diameter by up to 30%.[21,22] This mechanism of injury is thought to cause mechanical deformation of the cord, resulting in a transient increase in intracellular calcium concentrations.[17]

Athletes with cervical cord neuropraxia should initially be managed as if they have suffered a serious cervical injury. As noted earlier, this management includes spinal immobilization, transportation to the local emergency department for full neurologic evaluation, obtaining cervical spine radiographs (anteroposterior, lateral, and odontoid views), and performing cervical MRI. Return-to-play recommendations for athletes after cervical cord neuropraxia depend on multiple factors. An athlete who has sustained a single episode of neuropraxia with complete resolution of neurologic symptoms, no cervical spine laxity, normal radiographic results, and normal MRI results with no findings of functional spinal stenosis is thought by some experts to be safe to return to contact or collision sports.[17] Before return to contact sports, these athletes should be thoroughly evaluated by an expert practitioner to rule out functional stenosis or other conditions that may increase risk for spinal cord injury. Athletes with a single uncomplicated episode of neuropraxia with complete resolution of symptoms, but with significant spinal stenosis, intervertebral disk disease, or degenerative joint disease of the cervical spine, have a relative contraindication for participation in contact or collision sports. Athletes with an episode of cervical cord neuropraxia with cervical spine instability, neurologic symptoms lasting longer than 36 hours, MRI findings of spinal cord edema or injury, or bony abnormalities are contraindicated from participation in contact or collision sports.[17] Athletes with multiple episodes of cervical cord neuropraxia are contraindicated from participating in contact or collision sports.[17]

CERVICAL SPINAL STENOSIS

Several investigators have suggested a correlation between cervical spinal stenosis and cervical cord neuropraxia. However, the association between cervical spinal stenosis and the risk of permanent spinal cord injury during contact or collision sports remains controversial.[21] For levels C3-C7, normal spinal canals are at least 15 mm in anteroposterior diameter. Canals shorter than 13 mm in anteroposterior diameter are considered to be stenotic.[23] Torg, in 1986, and Pavlov, in 1987, designed a radiographic method to assess for cervical spinal stenosis using lateral cervical radiographs.[23] The Torg ratio (**Fig. 1**) is based on comparison between the sagittal diameters of the spinal canal and the middle of the vertebral body at the same level.

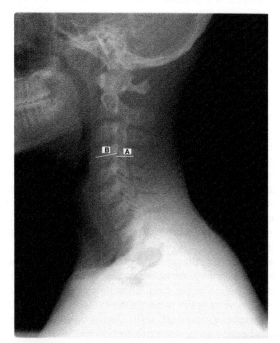

Fig. 1. The Torg ratio (A/B) is a comparison between the sagittal diameter of the spinal canal (A) and sagittal diameter of the vertebral body (B).

It has been suggested that a ratio less than 0.8 indicates significant spinal stenosis.[21] The Torg ratio may be clinically useful in counseling patients with prior episodes of cervical cord neuropraxia. Many investigators believe that athletes with a prior episode of cervical cord neuropraxia and a Torg ratio of less than 0.5 have approximately 75% risk of a future episode if cleared to return to contact or collision sports.[17]

However, Torg ratios are not recommended as screening tools in asymptomatic athletes. Subsequent studies have suggested that the Torg ratio is sensitive but has a low specificity and positive predictive value.[17] As such, using the Torg ratio as a screening tool potentially results in many false-positive results. It has been postulated that the high incidence of false-positives may be because of the large size of vertebral bodies of larger athletes. Many of these athletes have normal spinal canal diameters; however, the Torg ratio is potentially skewed by large vertebral body diameters. It has been recommended that athletes found to have an abnormal Torg ratio should undergo further workup before being diagnosed as having significant spinal stenosis.[23]

MRI has been proposed as a better method for assessing cervical spine stenosis. The common use of MRI in the assessment of cervical injury has led to the term functional spinal stenosis, which is defined as the obliteration of the local subarachnoid space containing cerebrospinal fluid with or without contour deformation of the cervical spinal cord.[23] Some experts believe that athletes with functional spinal stenosis have an increased risk of sustaining a severe spinal cord injury after head or neck trauma. These investigators have recommended that athletes who have a history of cervical cord neuropraxia and functional spinal stenosis be forbidden from participation in contact or collision sports.[23]

The recommendations for return to play in asymptomatic athletes with an episode of neuropraxia and known spinal stenosis are controversial. Torg recommends that asymptomatic athletes with a Torg ratio less than 0.8, absent cervical spine instability or structural defects, and normal radiographic results do not have an increased risk of cervical injury resulting in permanent neurologic damage. The investigator recommends that participation in contact or collision sports in this population of athletes should not be prohibited. On the other hand, Cantu[23] has concluded that athletes with cervical spinal stenosis have an increased risk of transient quadriparesis and permanent neurologic injury. He recommends that participation in contact or collision sports should be contraindicated.[21] Further studies are needed to better define the athletes at risk for future injury.

SPINAL CORD INJURY

There are several types of traumatic spinal cord lesions that can occur with sports-related cervical spine injury. The various types of traumatic spinal cord lesions include contusion (**Fig. 2**), edema, hemorrhage, and transection. Hemorrhage and transection of the spinal cord are considered irreversible and are thus heavily associated with complete spinal cord injury. Edema and contusion are thought to have more potential for neurologic recovery and are more heavily associated with incomplete injuries.[24] Most cases of tetraplegia in the absence of spinal stenosis result from a fracture dislocation in the cervical spine.[25] If a cervical fracture is suspected, the spine must be immobilized until either cervical spine injury has been ruled out or definitive stabilization has occurred.

The pathophysiology of acute spinal cord injury can be divided into primary and secondary phases. The primary phase occurs rapidly after the initial impact of injury, leading to mechanical damage, cell death, and severing of axons and vasculature.

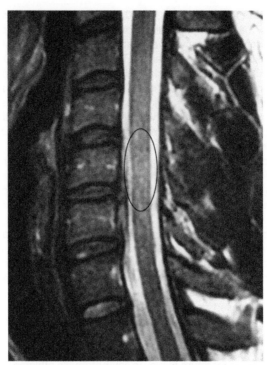

Fig. 2. A magnetic resonance image (sagittal) demonstrating spinal cord contusion (edema in central portion of spinal cord).

Secondary injury, as implied, is related to injury in the primary phase. Secondary injury occurs within several days, can last up to several months, and leads to irreversible damage to the spinal cord. Prevention of secondary injury is a topic of interest that is being investigated and is controversial. Although no interventions up to this point have been found efficacious in clinical trials, methylprednisolone is thought to have potential as an acute intervention. Methylprednisolone is theorized to reduce injury to the spinal cord by inhibiting lipid peroxidation, which stabilizes cell membranes, minimizing ischemia and reducing necrosis. Methylprednisolone has also been postulated to decrease interleukins, prostaglandins, and thromboxanes, which are mediators of inflammation.[26] Methylprednisolone can be used in patients with nonpenetrating spinal cord injuries and may be initiated up to 8 hours after injury.[26] Hypothermia is another intervention thought to have potential for prevention of secondary injury because hyperthermia has been shown in animal models to be detrimental to recovery. There are several anecdotal cases but little published scientific literature justifying the use of hypothermia in acute spinal cord injury. Complications of hypothermia include cardiac arrhythmias, coagulopathy, and increased incidence of infections.[26]

CERVICAL SPRAINS AND STRAINS

Once a severe cervical injury has been ruled out, the athlete can be evaluated for the presence of soft tissue injury, such as cervical strains or sprains. Both cervical strain and sprain are stretch injuries; cervical strains involve the cervical muscles or myotendinous junctions, whereas cervical sprains involve the cervical spine ligaments. There is often overlap between strains and sprains, such that both injuries often occur simultaneously during a single traumatic event.[27] Cervical strains often occur during an applied force to the head or neck during muscle contraction. The mechanism of injury causes an eccentric contraction leading to microscopic or gross tensile failure, most often at the myotendinous junction. Muscles with a high percentage of fast-twitch (type II) muscle fibers are at an increased risk of strain injuries.[27] Most cervical strains can be successfully managed conservatively with rest, ice, oral nonsteroidal antiinflammatory medications, muscle relaxants, gentle range of motion, and exercise. In some cases, manipulation by an osteopathic physician, a chiropractor, or a therapist can be helpful. Once the athlete has regained full range of motion and strength, return to contact sports is allowed.

Cervical sprains range from minor ligamentous injury with no laxity to gross ligament disruption with instability and dislocation. Cervical sprains often take longer to heal and, in more severe cases, can cause cervical laxity, leading to increased risk of sustaining neurologic injury. One of the most common mechanisms of cervical sprains is an acceleration-deceleration force applied to the neck. Ligament laxity is the most common concern when evaluating for a cervical sprain, thus it is imperative to avoid testing passive cervical range of motion. Active range of motion or gentle isometric contraction can be performed to help assess for laxity. If there is any concern for ligamentous laxity, immobilization of the cervical spine, radiographic assessment (including flexion and extension views), and evaluation by a spine specialist are warranted. Flexion and extension radiographs have been found to be a helpful additive to the traditional anteroposterior, lateral, and odontoid views when assessing for cervical laxity.[28] Anteroposterior displacement greater than 3.5 mm on flexion and extension views or 11° of rotation on anteroposterior radiographs is diagnostic of cervical ligament laxity. Athletes with these radiographic findings are prohibited from participation in contact or collision sports. Having laxity with less than 3.5 mm anteroposterior displacement on flexion and extension views or less than 11° of rotation on anteroposterior views is a relative contraindication to participation in contact or collision sports.[17] Minor cervical sprains can also be managed conservatively with rest, ice, oral nonsteroidal antiinflammatory medication, and gentle range of motion. Manipulation should be avoided in those with severe cervical pain or spasm and especially in cases of cervical laxity.

DISCOGENIC/RADICULAR PAIN

Cervical radiculopathy represents dysfunction of the cervical nerve root. The most commonly involved cervical nerve roots are C7 (60%) and C6 (25%).[28] The incidence of cervical radiculopathy in athletics is not well documented in the literature. Football and wrestling are thought by some to have an increased risk of cervical nerve root injury because of the high degree of contact and the potential for flexion, extension, and rotational cervical injuries, which can acutely compress the neuroforamina.[29] These motions are also a common mechanism for stinger injuries as described earlier.[29]

Weakness may be more noticeable to the athlete who participates in a sport requiring upper extremity strength. It is rare for a patient to have motor weakness without significant sensory or pain complaints. Any presentation of symptoms involving bilateral upper extremities more likely represents dysfunction of the spinal cord and should be evaluated for central canal stenosis.[29] Further details regarding presentation, imaging, electrodiagnosis, and treatment of cervical radiculopathy are discussed in other articles elsewhere in this issue. Although needle EMG can be helpful in the assessment of nerve root dysfunction, as mentioned earlier, electrodiagnostic abnormalities can persist for months to years after resolution of symptoms and thus are not helpful for determining return to play.[29] Athletes are cleared to return to sports once they have regained full strength and baseline range of motion, are asymptomatic, and have completed the necessary rehabilitation.[27]

Athletes who fail conservative management and continue to have focal neurologic symptoms or worsening signs and symptoms of radiculopathy should be evaluated by a spine surgeon. For athletes who have undergone surgery, return-to-play guidelines depend on the level of surgery and the number of spinal fusions. Athletes who have undergone a stable 1-level fusion at or below C3 are not contraindicated from returning to contact or collision sports. Asymptomatic athletes who have undergone 2- or 3-level spinal fusion may be able to return to contact or collision sports, although return is usually not advised because of the increased stresses placed on the vertebrae and disks adjacent to the levels of fusion and increased risk of degenerative changes. Athletes who have undergone spinal fusions above C3 and involving more than 3 spinal levels are prohibited from participation in contact or collision sports.[17]

UNIQUE POPULATIONS

Certain populations of patients are prone to structural anomalies, which place them at an increased risk of spinal cord injury during athletic participation. Patients with Down syndrome are of particular concern because 10% to 20% of these patients have atlantoaxial (AA) instability. AA instability is caused by laxity of the transverse ligament, which holds the dens of the axis in place on the inner aspect of the anterior arch of the atlas. This ligament assists in maintaining the integrity of the AA articulation.[30] Neurologic signs and symptoms tend to develop in up to 12% to 16% of patients with Down syndrome with such instability.[31]

For athletes competing in the Special Olympics, a complete preparticipation medical screening is necessary before clearance for competition. Radiographic imaging of the cervical spine is a mandatory component of the screening process for all athletes with Down syndrome who hope to participate in the Special Olympics.[19] Radiographs should include lateral views of the cervical spine in neutral, full flexion, and full extension. Athletes with abnormal radiographic results (atlantoodontoid distance >3.5 mm in adults or 5–6 mm in children) are restricted from contact events, such as diving, soccer, gymnastics, and floor hockey, and are limited to participation in noncontact sports, such as bowling, cross-country skiing, and distance running. There is some controversy regarding radiographic screening because some patients with normal radiographic results develop radiographic abnormalities as they age. There are also patients with radiographic evidence of AA instability, which becomes normal on follow-up radiographs.[19] Regardless, all patients with Down syndrome require radiographic clearance before Special Olympics participation.

Neurologic signs and symptoms of patients with Down syndrome with AA instability can vary. Typical findings include upper motor neuron signs, such as spasticity, brisk deep tendon reflexes, clonus, coordination deficits, and gait abnormalities. Neck pain, impaired cervical mobility, and torticollis are other common findings. Patients with any of these signs or symptoms should undergo a full workup, including MRI of the neck and evaluation by a specialist before being cleared for any sport. Patients with known AA instability, with or without unstable neurologic signs or symptoms, are often restricted from all contact sports, including football and wrestling.[19] Patients with AA instability and stable neurologic signs and symptoms should have recent

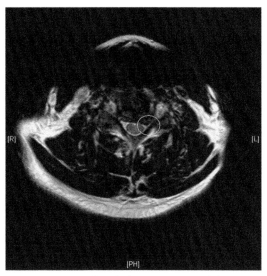

Fig. 3. A magnetic resonance image (axial) demonstrating a left cervical disk herniation.

radiographs before medical clearance in all athletic events, including noncontact sports (**Fig. 3**).

SUMMARY

It is essential for physicians evaluating cervical pain in the athlete to be able to distinguish between minor and severe cervical injuries. This distinction can be accomplished by having a thorough understanding of cervical anatomy, mechanisms of injury, and signs and symptoms of severe cervical spine injury. Conscious athletes can be more easily assessed on the field by history taking and physical examination, whereas unconscious athletes must be presumed to have a severe cervical spine injury until proven otherwise. Conscious athletes suspected of having a serious cervical injury and unconscious athletes should be managed with continuous monitoring of ABCs with jaw thrust maneuvers only for airway management, should have their helmet left in place with removal of the face mask, should be maintained in spinal immobilization, and should be transported to the local emergency department for further neurologic evaluation and imaging studies.

The goal of evaluating and managing cervical pain is to protect the athlete, which may involve either removing the athlete from the field of play or transporting the athlete to the emergency department for further evaluation. These decisions are often made by the covering physician on the sidelines. Having a basic understanding of cervical pain in the athlete is helpful for both the team physician and the office-based physician.

REFERENCES

1. Kraemer WJ, Torine JC, Silvestre R, et al. Body size and composition of National Football League players. J Strength Cond Res 2005;19(3):485–9.
2. Quinney HA, Dewart R, Game A, et al. A 26 year physiological description of a National Hockey League team. Appl Physiol Nutr Metab 2008;33(4):753–60.

3. Boden BP, Jarvis CG. Spinal injuries in sports. Phys Med Rehabil Clin N Am 2009; 20(1):55–68, vii.
4. Rihn JA, Anderson DT, Lamb K, et al. Cervical spine injuries in American football. Sports Med 2009;39(9):697–708.
5. Torg JS, Sennett B, Pavlov H, et al. Spear tackler's spine. An entity precluding participation in tackle football and collision activities that expose the cervical spine to axial energy inputs. Am J Sports Med 1993;21(5):640–9.
6. Torg JS, Truex R Jr, Quedenfeld TC, et al. The national football head and neck injury registry: report and conclusions 1978. JAMA 1979;241(14):1477–9.
7. Chao S, Pacella MJ, Torg JS. The pathomechanics, pathophysiology and prevention of cervical spinal cord and brachial plexus injuries in athletics. Sports Med 2010;40(1):59–75.
8. Waninger KN. On-field management of potential cervical spine injury in helmeted football players: leave the helmet on! Clin J Sport Med 1998;8(2):124–9.
9. Toler JD, Petschauer MA, Mihalik JP, et al. Comparison of 3 airway access techniques during suspected spine injury management in American football. Clin J Sport Med 2010;20(2):92–7.
10. Waninger KN. Management of the helmeted athlete with suspected cervical spine injury. Am J Sports Med 2004;32(5):1331–50.
11. Hoffman JR, Mower WR, Wolfson AB, et al. Validity of a set of clinical criteria to rule out injury to the cervical spine in patients with blunt trauma. N Engl J Med 2000;343(2):94–9.
12. Stiell IG, Clement CM, McKnight RD, et al. The Canadian C-spine rule for radiography in alert and stable trauma patients. JAMA 2001;286(15):1841–8.
13. Stiell IG, Clement CM, McKnight RD, et al. The Canadian C-spine rule versus the NEXUS low-risk criteria in patients with trauma. N Engl J Med 2003;349(26):2510–8.
14. Ghiselli D, Schaadt G, Mcallister DR. On-the-field evaluation of an athlete with a head or neck injury. Clin J Sport Med 2003;22:445–65.
15. Speer KP, Bassett FJ III. The prolonged burner syndrome. Am J Sports Med 1990;18(6):591–4.
16. Garrick JG, Web DR. Sports injuries: diagnosis and management. 2nd edition. Philadelphia: WB Saunders; 1999. p. 202–3.
17. Torg JS, Ramsey-Emrheim JA. Cervical spine and brachial plexus injuries: return to play recommendations. Phys Sportsmed 1997;25(7):61–88.
18. Gorden JA, Straub SJ, Swanik CB, et al. Effects of football collars on cervical hyperextension and lateral flexion. J Athl Train 2003;38(3):209–15.
19. Dorshimer GW, Kelly M. Cervical pain in the athlete: common conditions and treatment. Prim Care 2005;32:231–43.
20. Standaert CJ, Herring SA. Expert opinion and controversies in musculoskeletal and sports medicine: stingers. Arch Phys Med Rehabil 2009;90:402–6.
21. Allen CR, Kang JD. Transient quadriparesis in the athlete. Clin J Sport Med 2001; 21(1):16.
22. Moiel RH, Raso E, Waltz TA. Central cord syndrome resulting from congenital narrowness of the cervical spinal canal. J Trauma 1970;10:502–10.
23. Cantu RC. The cervical spinal stenosis controversy. Clin Sports Med 1998;17(1): 121–6.
24. Ramon S, Dominguez R, Ramirez L, et al. Clinical and magnetic resonance imaging correlation in acute spinal cord injury. Spinal Cord 1997;35(10):664–73.
25. Protcor MR, Cantu RC. Neck injuries. In: Frontera WR, Herring SA, Micheli LJ, et al, editors. Clinical Sports Medicine. Philadelphia: Saunders Elsevier; 2007. p. 142–313.

26. Walsh KA, Weant KA, Cook AM. Potential benefits of high-dose methylprednisolone in acute spinal cord injuries. Orthopedics 2010;33(4):249–52.
27. Zmurko MG, Tannoury TY, Tannoury CA, et al. Cervical sprains, disc herniations, minor fractures and other cervical injuries in the athlete. Clin Sports Med 2003;22: 513–21.
28. Murphey F, Simmons JC, Brunson B. Ruptured cervical discs. 1939–1972. Clin Neurosurg 1973;20(9):9–17.
29. Malanga G. The diagnosis and treatment of cervical radiculopathy. Med Sci Sports Exerc 1997;29(7):S236–45.
30. Pueschel SM, Scola FH, Perry CD, et al. Atlanto-axial instability in children with Down syndrome. Pediatr Radiol 1981;10(3):129–32.
31. Winell J, Burke SW. Sports participation of children with Down syndrome. Orthop Clin North Am 2003;34:440.

Thoracic Outlet Syndrome

Glenn Ozoa, DO[a],*, Daniel Alves, MD[b], David E. Fish, MD, MPH[c,d]

KEYWORDS

- Thoracic outlet syndrome • Neurogenic TOS • Vascular TOS
- Disputed TOS • Interscalene triangle • Costoclavicular triangle
- Subpectorialis minor space

Of the many clinical entities involving the neck region, one of the most intriguing is thoracic outlet syndrome (TOS). TOS is an array of disorders that involves injury to the neurovascular structures in the cervicobrachial region. A classification system based on etiology, symptoms, clinical presentation, and anatomy is supported by most physicians. The first type of TOS is vascular, involving compression of either the subclavian artery or vein. The second type is true neurogenic TOS, which involves injury to the brachial plexus. Finally, the third and most controversial type is referred to as disputed neurogenic TOS. This article aims to provide the reader some understanding of the pathophysiology, workup, and treatment of this fascinating clinical entity.

PATHOANATOMY

There are 3 common locations for compression of the neurovascular bundle in TOS: the interscalene triangle, the costoclavicular space, and the subpectorialis minor space (**Fig. 1**).

The interscalene triangle is formed by the first rib and the anterior and middle scalene muscles (see **Fig. 1**). Traveling through this space are the trunks of the brachial plexus along with the subclavian artery. There are a number of potential anatomic anomalies in this region that can cause injury to the neurovascular bundle. These structural aberrations include cervical ribs, fibrous bands, rib anomalies, callus formations, tumor, and scalene muscle insertion variation.[1] It has been postulated that congenital soft tissue anomalies in the thoracic outlet region are common and remain

The authors have nothing to disclose.

[a] Beverly Hills Orthopedic Group, 120 South Spalding Drive, Suite 401, Beverly Hills, CA 90212, USA

[b] Universal Pain Management, Los Angeles, CA, USA

[c] Division of Interventional Physiatry, Physical Medicine and Rehabiliation, The UCLA Spine Center, David Geffen School of Medicine at UCLA, Los Angeles, CA, USA

[d] Department of Orthopaedics, Physical Medicine and Rehabiliation, The UCLA Spine Center, David Geffen School of Medicine at UCLA, Los Angeles, CA, USA

* Corresponding author.

E-mail address: gozoa@bhorthogroup.com

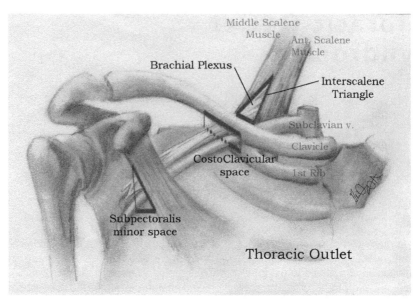

Fig. 1. Thoracic outlet anatomy. (*Courtesy of* Glenn Ozoa, DO.)

symptomatically quiescent until a triggering action prompts these variations into a pathologic state. This action can be in the form of a sudden traumatic event such as a motor vehicle accident, which can cause spasm of the scalene musculature. The inciting cause can also be more gradual, such as from occupational or athletic activities that promote muscular hypertrophy or imbalances.[2,3]

The costoclavicular space is the second area where compression can occur. It is a triangular region generally located between the clavicle and first rib (see **Fig. 1**). In this region, compressive injury to the neurovascular bundle can be caused by a number of congenital or acquired abnormalities involving the rib, clavicle, subclavian muscle, or costocoracoid ligament. For example, persons with postural issues such as drooping shoulders from deconditioning, a large pendulous breast, or heavy backpack carriage are believed to have a narrower costoclavicular space that may make them susceptible to TOS.[1,4,5]

The third location is a region below the coracoid process just under the pectoralis minor tendon. This is referred to as the subpectoralis minor space or the subcoracoid space (see **Fig. 1**). It is believed that compression through this space can occur via mechanisms associated with arm abduction, in which the neurovascular bundle gets stressed underneath a taut pectoralis minor tendon. This positional injury to the neurovascular tissue was first referred to as hyperabduction syndrome by Wright in 1945. It is believed to be observed typically in stocky, short, muscular males who have occupations associated with prolonged overhead activities (**Fig. 2**).[1,6]

EPIDEMIOLOGY

Historically, the diagnosis of TOS has been controversial. Consequently, the prevalence of this condition has been poorly documented. The incidences of true neurogenic TOS and vascular TOS have been estimated in some reports to be as rare as 1 case per 1 million people.[7] Disputed neurogenic TOS is more prevalent, and the overall incidence of this form of TOS is reported to range from 3 to 80 per 1000 people.

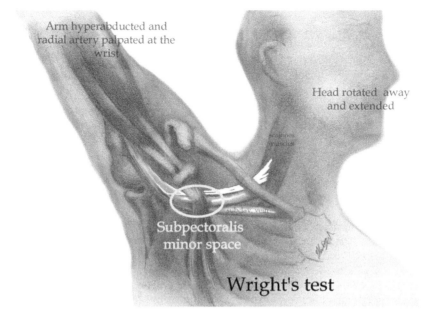

Arm hyperabducted and radial artery palpated at the wrist

Head rotated away and extended

scalene muscles

subclavian vein

Subpectoralis minor space

Wright's test

Fig. 2. The hyperabduction test or Wright test. (*Courtesy of* Glenn Ozoa, DO.)

The age of onset is typically between 20 and 40 years and overall TOS is reported to be more common in women than men.[8,9]

CLINICAL PRESENTATIONS
Arterial TOS

Arterial TOS is reported to account for 1% to 5% of all TOS cases.[10] This form of TOS is the result of compression of the subclavian artery in the region of the interscalene triangle.[11] In a retrospective study of 50 cases of arterial TOS, Durham and colleagues[12] found that the causative factor in most cases was a bony anomaly such as a cervical or anomalous first rib. The patient with arterial TOS may complain of intermittent arm pain, paresthesia, and fatigability with use or overhead positioning. Additionally, there may be findings of weakness, coolness, pallor, and diminished pulse in the affected extremity. In severe arterial TOS, vessel damage could result in poststenotic aneurysm or distal embolic occlusions causing advanced ischemic damage to the extremity. As such, this makes arterial TOS the most threatening form of the syndrome.[3,10,11,13]

Venous TOS

Venous TOS represents 2% to 3% of all forms of TOS.[10] Venous TOS typically results from compressive injury to the subclavian and/or axillary vein in the costoclavicular space.[10,14–16] Compromise to the vascular structures can occur via 2 mechanisms: (1) a positional compression of the vein between the clavicle and first rib with overhead activities; or (2) repeated friction between the vein and clavicle, which triggers an intra-vascular thrombotic mechanism.[17] Moreover, the clinical manifestations vary based on the mechanism of vascular insult. In patients with positional compression, an inter-mittent uncomfortable heaviness and swelling of the affected arm may be reported with overhead use. Patients with symptoms resulting from thrombosis may have pain along the course of the axillary vein with edema and cyanosis in the upper extremity associated with distended collateral superficial veins in the shoulder and anterior chest.[16,18,19] Serious complications of advanced venous thrombosis are pulmonary embolus, severe pain, and edema.

Neurogenic TOS

Accounting for 90% to 97% of TOS cases, the neurogenic type has been subdivided into "true" neurogenic TOS (N-TOS), and more common "disputed" neurogenic TOS.[20] Both forms are secondary to compressive or traction injury typically to the lower trunk of the brachial plexus.[19] True neurogenic TOS has earned the "true" designation owing to anatomic and electrodiagnostic evidence that supports the diagnosis. In contrast, the "disputed" neurogenic TOS, also known as common or nonspecific TOS, is believed by many to be a vague clinical entity lacking any objective clinical findings.[21]

The classical form of true neurogenic TOS is called Gilliatt-Summer Hand.[22,23] This syndrome was first described in 1970 as thenar, hypothenar, and interossei weakness and/or atrophy, plus ulnar and medial antebrachial cutaneous hypoesthesia in the affected arm. Patients with true neurogenic TOS may report an array of symptoms involving pain, numbness, paresthesia, and weakness in the upper extremity. Aggravating activities may be overhead arm maneuvers and lifting heavy objects.

Approximately 85% of patients diagnosed with TOS are thought to have the disputed type. This form of TOS is reportedly associated with an ill-defined and inconsistent symptomatology in the absence of confirming objective evidence.[21] Therefore, it has been shrouded in controversy, with a number of physicians questioning its very existence.[8,24] Patients with disputed neurogenic TOS will have similar complaints of paresthesia and weakness as those with neurogenic TOS. However, there usually are more complaints of pain. Additionally, there may be other symptoms more proximal to the thoracic outlet such as vision/hearing disturbances, headaches, and facial pain. This myriad of symptoms is thought to be a result of the variability between upper versus lower compression sites of the brachial plexus.[1] Triggering factors are thought to be repetitive motion disorders, postural issues, or traumatic movements of the neck or shoulder that can cause dysfunction to the scalene musculature.

DIAGNOSIS

The workup for TOS begins with a thorough history, with attention to any trauma to the shoulder or neck region. Any occupational or athletic activities that involve prolonged use of the upper extremities in awkward positions should be appreciated.[2] One must also be mindful of the differential diagnosis of upper extremity pain, weakness, and sensation changes.

The physical examination is crucial to the diagnosis of TOS. During visual inspection of the cervical region, an assessment of muscle asymmetry, deformities, and posture should be noted. A careful comparison between the upper extremities should be made with attention to atrophy, color, edema, moisture, and hair growth.

Other important aspects of the examination include palpation for tenderness, texture changes, masses, or vascular pulsations in the cervicothoracic region. Additionally, finger pressure or percussion should be applied to the supraclavicular fossa to determine if symptoms distally in the arm can be elicited. Finally, a thorough neurologic examination of the cervical spine and upper extremities, including range of motion and strength testing, should be performed.

There are a number of provocative tests that may assist in the diagnosis of TOS. By mechanically stressing specific regions between the neck and shoulder, these physical maneuvers are intended to cause temporary neurologic or vascular derangement. However, the sensitivity and specificity of these tests is relatively low.[25]

In the Adson test, the interscalene space is thought to be stressed. In this test (**Fig. 3**), the patient is sitting, with the examiner's fingers placed over the radial artery. The patient's arm is then externally rotated and extended while palpating the radial pulse. The patient then extends and rotates the neck toward the test arm and takes a deep breath. The production of an absent or diminished radial pulse is suggestive of compression of the subclavian artery by the scalene muscles.[9,25,26]

Another provocative maneuver to determine vascular compromise is the Allen test. The patient is seated with the test shoulder placed in 90 degrees of abduction and external rotation, and the elbow in 90 degrees of flexion. The examiner stands with his or her fingers over the radial artery at the wrist. As the patient rotates the neck away from the test arm the examiner palpates the radial pulse. An absent or diminished radial pulse is suggestive of TOS.[9,25,26]

To test for impingement at the costoclavicular region, the military brace test (**Fig. 4**) can be used. With the patient standing at rest, the patient is asked to retract and

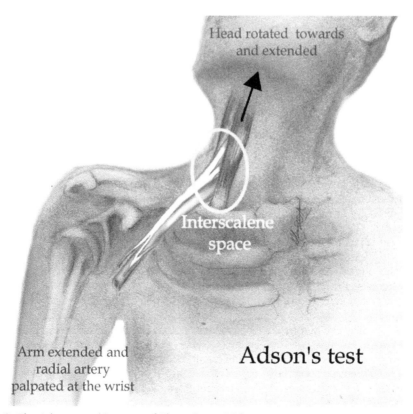

Fig. 3. The Adson test. (*Courtesy of* Glenn Ozoa, DO.)

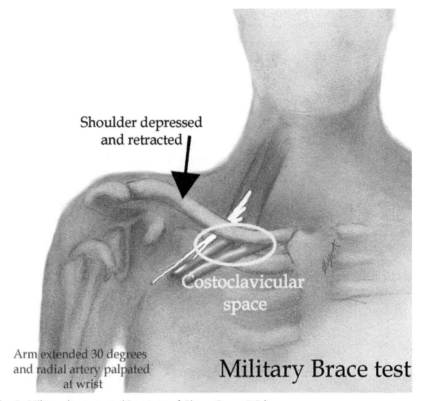

Fig. 4. Military brace test. (*Courtesy of* Glenn Ozoa, DO.)

depress the shoulders. The humerus is then extended 30 degrees with the neck hyper-extended. In this position the space between the clavicle and first rib diminishes. If the radial pulse disappears, this suggests impingement of the subclavian artery at the costoclavicular region.[9,25,26]

The elevated arm stress test, or Roos test, theoretically examines both neural and vascular components. It is performed by having the patient sit or stand with both shoulders in 90 degrees of abduction and external rotation, and the elbows in 90 degrees of flexion. The patient is then asked to open and close both hands for 3 minutes. The patient with TOS may have the inability to maintain this test position because of pain or sensory/motor disturbances.[9,25,26]

In the hyperabduction or Wright test (see **Fig. 2**), the neurovascular bundle is stressed underneath the pectoralis minor tendon. In this test, the patient's arm is hyperabducted through shoulder external rotation and abduction while the radial pulse is palpated. A diminished pulse and reproduction of paresthesias is considered positive.[9,25,26]

The reliability and purpose of these maneuvers has been a matter of contention. For example, in one study of 100 healthy,[27] it was found that the Adson maneuver had a false-positive rate of 13.5% and the hyperabduction test had a false-positive rate of 57%. Moreover, some have argued that these maneuvers could provoke carpal or cubital tunnel symptoms.[28] Given this controversy, these provocative tests should be considered in conjunction with the history, physical examination, and other ancillary testing to most effectively guide the diagnosis.

ANCILLARY TESTING

In the evaluation of TOS, imaging studies may be helpful. Plain radiographs of the cervical spine and chest can reveal the presence of congenital or acquired bony abnormalities such as cervical ribs, C7 transversomegaly, healed fractures, rib anomalies, and degenerative arthritic changes. Also, the overall carriage of the shoulder girdle can be evaluated with attention to the costoclavicular space.[4]

To visualize finer anatomic details, magnetic resonance imaging (MRI) and/or computed tomography (CT) can be used. With these studies the intricate relationships between the bony anatomy and soft tissue can be appreciated. However, these imaging studies are more useful in evaluating other conditions, such as masses in the cervicothoracic region or degenerative disease of the cervical spine. Moreover, the use of static imaging to study TOS is thought to be problematic because the compromise to the neurovascular bundle can be a positional phenomenon. As such, alternative imaging methods that incorporate dynamic positioning, such as MRI or spiral CT, have been explored.[29,30]

Currently, most physicians consider conventional arteriography or venography the most reliable test for evaluating symptoms of arterial or venous compromise in thoracic outlet syndrome.[11,16] However, recent studies have shown that CT and MR angiography may serve as promising alternatives.[31,32]

The arterial and venous system of the thoracic outlet have also been studied using duplex ultrasonography. Demondion and colleagues[33] demonstrated that B-mode in color duplex ultrasonography study with postural maneuvers is a good supplementary imaging device to CT and MR imaging. On the other hand, studying the venous systems with duplex scanning is thought to generate a high false-positive rate because the clavicle obstructs the view of the subclavian vein, and a high false-negative rate from the presence of large collaterals.[16]

A relatively new imaging technique in evaluating TOS is MR neurography. This imaging protocol reportedly allows visualization of nerve swelling, mechanical deviations in nerve path, and nervous tissue hyperdensities suggestive of injury.[34] Filler and colleagues[35] demonstrated that application of MR neurography to thoracic outlet syndrome could potentially have remarkable clinical significance.

Electrodiagnostic Studies

Nerve conduction studies (NCS) and electromyography (EMG) can be helpful in providing electrodiagnostic evidence to support neurogenic TOS and to rule out other etiologies such as cervical radiculopathy or distal nerve entrapment neuropathies.[21] In true neurogenic TOS, the lower trunk of the brachial plexus, composed of C8-T1, is the most affected. Nerve conduction studies may reveal the following: decreased amplitude or unobtainable ulnar and medial antebrachial cutaneous sensory nerve action potentials (SNAP) and decreased amplitude in median nerve compound motor action potentials (CMAP). Notably, because the median nerve's sensory component is derived from the upper trunk, median SNAPs are normal. Moreover, the presence of an abnormal ulnar SNAP suggests that the lesion is not at the level of the intraspinal canal, which is evidence against a cervical radiculopathy or myelopathy.[36–39]

During needle electrode examination, muscles innervated by the C8-T1 roots or lower trunk should be assessed. The abductor pollicis brevis is the most affected muscle, followed by the intrinsic muscles of the hand. In the more contentious, disputed N-TOS, the role of electrodiagnostic testing is unclear. Additionally, the use of F-waves and somatosensory evoked potentials (SEPs) continue to remain controversial.[40,41]

Conservative Treatment of Neurogenic TOS

Patients with neurogenic TOS can be successfully treated with conservative measures, such as patient education, activity modifications, medications, and rehabilitative exercises promoting good posture and body mechanics control. Emphasis should be placed on the avoidance of exacerbating activities and removal of ergonomic stressors. Additionally, knowledge of specific aggravating factors can be instrumental in customizing a physical therapy program best suited for the patient.

It is important to address postural faults that may provoke or aggravate the symptoms of TOS. For example, these patients may exhibit a thoracic kyphosis associated with an anteriorly positioned head and protracted shoulders. In this situation, shortened scalene muscles and elongation of other neck muscles may position certain muscles of the cervicothoracic region at a mechanical disadvantage. Moreover, abnormal scapular movements in this setting further perpetuate weakness of the trapezius and serratus anterior muscle groups.[42,43]

In most cases of TOS, the primary targets of rehabilitative exercises are the scalene muscles; however, it is important to treat the upper trapezius, levator scapulae, sternocleiodomastoid, pectoral, and suboccipital muscles as well. Moreover, these muscles and any associated dysfunctions can be addressed with mobilization, muscle energy, and manipulative techniques used by osteopathic physicians, chiropractors, or physical therapists.[44]

At times, a myofascial pain syndrome can concomitantly exist with TOS as a result of compensatory body mechanics. Therefore, trigger points may be present. These tender and taut bands of muscle can be injected with local anesthetic and steroid solutions to provide relief and further promote the rehabilitative process.

In cases of neurogenic TOS unresponsive to the previously stated conservative measures, a more invasive approach to managing the condition can be used.[45] Jordan and colleagues found that the scalene muscles can be injected with an anesthetic or Botulinum toxin type A (Botox) with temporary improvement.[46–48] Furthermore, these researchers also found a 94% success rate with surgical decompression in those patients who benefited from scalene botox injections.[49]

Treatment of Vascular TOS

The management of vascular TOS is more aggressive than neurogenic TOS. In the rare suspected case of vascular TOS, consultation with a vascular surgeon should be the initial step in management. Emergency surgery is indicated in only extremely unusual instances, such as a patient with infarction caused by vascular occlusion or recurrent embolism.

SURGICAL MANAGEMENT

The indications for surgical management of TOS have been controversial. There is general consensus that acute arterial compromise warrants surgery.[50] However, for neurogenic and venous TOS, the indications for surgery are unclear. Some believe that progressive neurologic dysfunction or pain associated with functional impairment recalcitrant to 4 to 6 months of conservative management are reasons to consider surgery.[20,51]

The objective of most surgical procedures involves the release of the anterior and middle scalene muscles with possible resection of the first and/or cervical rib.[51] Two of the most common surgical approaches are via the transaxillary and the anterior supraclavicular spaces.[8,18,52,53] Unfortunately, the long-term surgical outcomes for

TOS have historically been inconsistent and contentious, particularly for disputed neurogenic TOS.[54–57]

SUMMARY

Thoracic outlet syndrome is a complex clinical entity. Diagnosis demands a sound knowledge of neuromuscular and vascular relationships in the neck region along with perceptive clinical skills. Also, attention to the differential diagnosis of other syndromes causing similar neck and arm symptoms must be carefully considered and ruled out.

REFERENCES

1. Atasoy E. Thoracic outlet syndrome: anatomy. Hand Clin 2004;20:7–14.
2. Nichols AW. The thoracic outlet syndrome in athletes. J Am Board Fam Pract 1996;9:346–55.
3. Roos DB. Thoracic outlet syndrome is underdiagnosed. Muscle Nerve 1999;22: 126–9.
4. Brantigan CO, Roos DB. Diagnosing thoracic outlet syndrome. Hand Clin 2004; 20:27–36.
5. Sanders RJ, Hammond SL. Etiology and pathology. Hand Clin 2004;20:23–6.
6. Wright IS. The neurovascular syndrome produced by hyperabduction of the arms: the immediate changes produced in 15 normal controls, and the effects on some persons of prolonged hyperabduction of the arms, as in sleeping, and certain occupations. Am Heart J 1945;29:1.
7. Ferrante MA. Brachial plexopathies: classification, causes, and consequences. Muscle Nerve 2004;30:547–68.
8. Huang JH, Zager EL. Thoracic outlet syndrome. Neurosurgery 2004;55:897–903.
9. Leffert RD. Thoracic outlet syndrome and the shoulder. Clin Sports Med 1983;2: 439–52.
10. Vanti C, Natalini L, Romeo A, et al. Conservative treatment of thoracic outlet syndrome. Eur Med Phys 2006;42:1–14.
11. Patton GM. Arterial thoracic outlet syndrome. Hand Clin 2004;20:107–11.
12. Durham JR, Yao JS, Pearce WH, et al. Arterial injuries in the thoracic outlet syndrome. J Vasc Surg 1995;21:57–69.
13. Sheth RN, Belzberg AJ. Diagnosis and treatment of thoracic outlet syndrome. Neurosurg Clin North Am 2001;12:295–309.
14. Becker F, Terriat B. [Thoracic outlet syndromes: the viewpoint of the angiologist]. Rev Med Interne 1999;20(Suppl 5):487S–93S [in French].
15. Holtzhausen LM, Matley P, de Jager W, et al. Extravascular axillary vein compression in a competitive swimmer: a case report. Clin J Sport Med 1995;5:129–33.
16. Sanders RJ, Hammond SL. Venous thoracic outlet syndrome. Hand Clin 2004;20: 113–8.
17. Coon WW, Willis PW 3rd. Thrombosis of axillary and subclavian veins. Arch Surg 1967;94:657–63.
18. Hughes ES. Venous obstruction in the upper extremity (Paget-Schroetter syndrome). Coll Rev 1949;88:89–127.
19. Karas SE. Thoracic outlet syndrome. Clin Sports Med 1990;9:297–310.
20. Silver D. Thoracic outlet syndrome. In: Sabiston DC, editor. Textbook of surgery: the biological basis of modern surgical practice. 13th edition. Philadelphia: WB Saunders Company; 1986. p. 1858.

21. Wilbourn AJ. Thoracic outlet syndrome is overdiagnosed. Muscle Nerve 1999;22: 130–8.
22. Gilliatt RW. Thoracic outlet syndromes. In: Bunge R, editor, Peripheral neuropathy, vol. 2. Philadelphia: WB Sanders; 1984. p. 1409–19.
23. Gilliatt RW, Le Quesne PM, Logue V, et al. Wasting of the hand associated with a cervical rib or band. J Neurol Neurosurg Psychiatry 1970;33:615–24.
24. Axelrod D, Proctor M, Geisser M, et al. Outcomes after surgery for thoracic outlet syndrome. J Vasc Surg 2001;33:1220–5.
25. Rayan GM, Jensen C. Thoracic outlet syndrome: provocative examination maneuvers in a typical population. J Shoulder Elbow Surg 1995;4:113–7.
26. Rayan GM. Thoracic outlet syndrome. J Shoulder Elbow Surg 1998;7:440–51.
27. Novak CB. Thoracic outlet syndrome. Clin Plast Surg 2003;30(2):175–88.
28. Naidu SH, Kothari MJ. Thoracic outlet syndrome: does fiction outweigh facts? Curr Opin Orthop 2003;12:209–14.
29. Demondion X, Bacqueville E, Paul C, et al. Thoracic outlet: assessment with MR imaging in asymptomatic and symptomatic populations. Radiology 2003;227: 461–8.
30. Remy-Jardin M, Doyen J, Remy J, et al. Functional anatomy of the thoracic outlet: evaluation with helical CT. Radiology 1997;205:843–51.
31. Dymarkowski S, Bosmans H, Marchal G. Three-dimensional MR angiography in the evaluation of thoracic outlet syndrome. AJR Am J Roentgenol 1999;173(4): 1005–8.
32. Remy-Jardin M, Remy J, Masson P. CT angiography of thoracic outlet syndrome: evaluation of imaging protocols for the detection of arterial stenosis. J Comput Assist Tomogr 2000;24(3):349–61.
33. Demondion X, Herbinet P, Van Sint Jan S, et al. B-mode and color duplex ultra-sonography (US) are good supplementary tools for assessment of vessel compression in association with postural maneuvers, especially in cases with positive clinical features of TOS but negative features of TOS at CT and MR imaging. Radiographics 2006;26:1735–50.
34. Filler AG, Kliot M, Howe FA, et al. Application of magnetic resonance neurography in the evaluation of patients with peripheral nerve pathology. Neurosurg 1996;85:299–309.
35. Filler AG, Maravilla KR, Tsuruda JS. MR neurography and muscle MR imaging for image diagnosis or disorders affecting the peripheral nerves and musculature. Neurol Clin 2004;22:643–82.
36. Cruz–Martinez A, Arpa J. Electrophysiological assessment in neurogenic thoracic outlet syndrome. Electromyogr Clin Neurophysiol 2001;41:253–6.
37. England JD, Tiel RL. AAEM case report 33: costoclavicular mass syndrome. American Association of Electrodiagnostic Medicine. Muscle Nerve 1999;22(3): 412–8.
38. Ferrante MA, Wilbourn AJ. The utility of various sensory nerve conduction responses in assessing brachial pleopathies. Muscle Nerve 1995;18:879–89.
39. Wilbourn AJ. Thoracic outlet syndromes. Neurol Clin 1999;17:477–97.
40. Aminoff MJ, Olney RK, Parry GJ, et al. Relative utility of different electrophysio-logic techniques in evaluation of brachial plexopathies. Neurology 1988;38: 546–50.
41. Komanetsky RM, Novak CB, MacKinnon SE. Somatosensory evoked potentials fail to diagnose thoracic outlet syndrome. J Hand Surg Am 1996;21:662–6.
42. Crosby CA, Wehbe MA. Conservative treatment for thoracic outlet syndrome. Hand Clin 2004;20:43–9.

43. Mackinnon SE, Novak CB. Thoracic outlet syndrome. Curr Probl Surg 2002;39: 1070–145.
44. Dobrusin R. An osteopathic approach to conservative management of thoracic outlet syndromes. J Am Osteopath Assoc 1989;89:1046–50, 1053–7.
45. Smith HS, Audette J, Royal MA. Botulinum toxin in pain management of soft tissue syndromes. Clin J Pain 2002;18(6):S147–54.
46. Cui M, Khanijou S, Rubino J, et al. Subcutaneous administration of botulinum toxin A reduces formalin-induced pain. Pain 2004;107:125–33.
47. Jordan SE, Machleder HI. Diagnosis of thoracic outlet syndrome using electrophysiologically guided anterior scalene blocks. Ann Vasc Surg 1998;12:260–4.
48. Jordan SE, Ahn SS, Freishlag JA, et al. Selective botulinum chemodenervation of the scalene muscles for treatment of neurogenic thoracic outlet syndrome. Ann Vasc Surg 2000;14:365–9.
49. Jamieson WG, Chinnick B. Thoracic outlet syndrome: fact or fancy? A review of 409 consecutive patients who underwent operation. Can J Surg 1996;39:321–6.
50. Kenny RA, Traynor GB, Withington D, et al. Thoracic outlet syndrome: a useful exercise treatment option. Am J Surg 1993;165:282–4.
51. Adson AW. Surgical treatment for symptoms produced by cervical ribs and the scalenus anticus muscle. 1947. Clin Orthop 1986;207:3–12.
52. Roos DB. The place for scalenectomy and first-rib resection in thoracic outlet syndrome. Surgery 1982;92:1077–85.
53. Cikrit DF, Haefner R, Nichols WK, et al. Transaxillary or supraclavicular decompression for the thoracic outlet syndrome. A comparison of the risk and benefits. Am Surg 1989;55:347–52.
54. Colli BO, Carlotti CG, Assirati JA, et al. Neurogenic thoracic outlet syndromes: a comparison of true and nonspecific syndromes after surgical treatment. Surg Neurol 2006;65:262–72.
55. Degeorges R, Reynaud C, Becquemin JP. Thoracic outlet syndrome surgery: long-term functional results. Ann Vasc Surg 2004;18:558–65.
56. Landry GJ, Moneta GL, Lloyd M, et al. Long-term functional outcome of neurogenic thoracic outlet syndrome in surgically and conservatively treated patients. J Vasc Surg 2001;33:312–9.
57. Povlsen B, Belzberg A, Hansson T, et al. Treatment for thoracic outlet syndrome. Cochrane Database Syst Rev 2010;1:CD007218.

Neck Pain from a Rheumatologic Perspective

Elana M. Oberstein, MD, MPH[a],*, Maria Carpintero, MD[b],
Aviva Hopkins, MD[b]

KEYWORDS

- Rheumatoid arthritis • Ankylosing spondylitis
- Diffuse idiopathic skeletal hyperostosis • Myositis
- Fibromyalgia

This article provides a comprehensive review of rheumatologic considerations for a clinician when evaluating a patient with neck pain. Clearly, anatomic derangements of the cervical spine should be considered when a patient complains of cervicalgia. However, one must also entertain the possibility of a systemic illness as the cause of the pain. Examples of diseases that may present with a prominent feature of neck pain are discussed. Evidence of an underlying rheumatic illness may guide the clinician in a different therapeutic direction.

RHEUMATOID ARTHRITIS

Rheumatoid arthritis (RA) is a systemic autoimmune disease, characterized by chronic inflammatory synovitis that affects 1% to 2% of the population. Typically, females are affected three times more often than males in the second to fourth decades of life. The pathogenesis of RA is not well understood but it is believed that an autoimmune inflammatory response against the synovium is triggered by an unknown risk factor in a genetically susceptible individual. RA is the most common inflammatory arthritis affecting the cervical spine,[1] affecting 17% to 84%[2,3] of patients with RA. However, only a minority of these patients develop neurologic complications.[4] The involvement and severity of cervical spine disease correlates with peripheral joint erosions, active synovitis, high levels of C-reactive protein (CRP), rheumatoid factor positivity, rheumatoid nodules, and age of onset of RA.[5] Symptoms usually develop with disease

The authors have nothing to disclose.

[a] Arthritis and Rheumatic Disease Specialties, 21097 NE 27th Court, Suite 200, Aventura, FL 33180, USA

[b] Divison of Rheumatology, Department of Internal Medicine, University of Miami Miller School of Medicine, 1120 NW 14th Street, Room 973, D4-10, Miami, FL 33136, USA

* Corresponding author.

E-mail address: eoberstein@med.miami.edu

duration of 10 or more years but patients with severe disease may develop symptoms within 2 years.[2]

In the cervical spine, it is believed that extension of the inflammatory process from the neurocentral joints results in ligamentous rupture, apophyseal joint erosions, and disc herniation with subsequent instability and subluxation.[6] Bursal proliferation is also involved in erosive changes. Although any cervical segment can be affected, the occipitoatlantoaxial junction is the most commonly affected due to the purely synovial characteristics of this joint.[5]

Atlantoaxial subluxation is the most common lesion affecting up to 86% of patients with RA.[1,5] Anterior movement of the axis is the most common type due to laxity and destruction of the transverse ligament. Pannus formation is also found in the odontoid region, and is associated with fractures and erosions of the odontoid process. Posterior subluxation, also associated with odontoid erosions or fractures, is less common. Destruction of the lateral atlantoaxial joints around the foramen magnum increases vertical movements in relation to the axis. Basilar invagination can occur in 5% to 32%[2] of patients and is secondary to inflammatory destruction of cartilage and bone from the occipitoatlantal and atlantoaxial joints. This allows the skull to descend on the cervical spine and an eroded odontoid can enter the foramen magnum, causing brain stem or cord compression, or sudden death. Subaxial subluxation is a late complication that develops as a result of destruction of multiple facet joints, the interspinous ligament, and the discovertebral junction at multiple levels giving a characteristic staircase appearance. This usually develops late in the disease course and is observed in up to 25% of patients with RA.[2]

Clinical Findings

Patients may be asymptomatic.[2] Presenting symptoms may vary depending on the affected level. Pain is the most common manifestation, present in up to 80% of patients.[2,6] Pain may radiate to the occipital, retro-orbital or temporal area with or without muscle spasm. Neurologic symptoms can include radicular pain and/or weakness, myelopathy with sensory and motor deficits, abnormal reflexes, or spasticity. C1-C2 subluxation is associated with medullary dysfunction such as respiratory irregularities, loss of consciousness, bladder or bowel incontinence, vertigo, or convulsions.[5] Patients presenting with vertebrobasilar insufficiency may have tinnitus, vertigo, loss of equilibrium, and gait abnormalities. On physical examination, patients may have loss of cervical spine lordosis, resistance to passive motion, and abnormal protrusion in the posterior pharyngeal wall. The most common neurologic findings are increased reflexes with abnormal plantar responses, weakness with muscle atrophy, spasticity, and gait disorders. Patients with severe disease have a poor prognosis without surgery and a high mortality rate.

Imaging

Routine screening among patients with RA includes anteroposterior, lateral, open mouth, and flexion-extension radiograph series. Screening should be done in all patients undergoing general anesthesia to evaluate for instability. Subsequent assessments are recommended every 2 to 3 years or if new symptoms develop.[5,7] Odontoid erosions, subaxial subluxations, apophyseal joint erosions, and disc narrowing are frequently seen.

Atlantoaxial subluxation showing a displacement of greater than 3 mm between C1 and the odontoid peg in flexion-extension films is considered abnormal. Separation between C1-C2 of more than 9 mm or a posterior atlantodental distance (PADI) of less than 14 mm are associated with increased risk for cord compression.[5] Subaxial subluxation is characterized by sequential vertebral listhesis with joint erosions and spinous process changes.

CT scan imaging may be helpful to assess erosive disease and cord compressions in patients with advanced disease and anatomic variations, but its use has been limited due to MRI technology. MRI is the diagnostic modality of choice; it permits a complete assessment of the cervical spine allowing visualization of pannus, ligaments, spinal cord, and bone. It detects the presence of erosive changes and the extension of the inflammatory process.[4,8] MRI should be performed in all patients with neurologic symptoms,[5] a PADI of less than 14 mm, or evidence of odontoid migration on plain films.

Treatment

Early and aggressive treatment of RA is thought to slow the progression of cervical spine involvement, but there is limited data supporting disease-modifying antirheumatic drug (DMARD) therapy for the prevention of cervical spine subluxation.[9,10] In patients with pain but no neurologic deficits, a cervical collar may provide support.[2] Anti-inflammatories, trigger point injections, and nerve blocks can provide temporary analgesia. Neither neck muscle strengthening exercises[11] nor heat therapy has demonstrated benefits. Manipulation of the neck should be avoided.

Early operative treatment in patients with subluxation and signs of spinal cord compression may delay the development of further complications, including death.[12,13] Other indications for surgical treatment include intractable pain, instability, myelopathy, vertebral artery compromise, PADI of less than14 mm on imaging, and neurologic deficits.[1] Operative options include decompression, laminectomy, foraminotomy, and fusion of the spine.[6] The most common surgical procedure for this condition is C1-C2 fusion followed by occipitocervical fusion. Surgery is usually well tolerated and improvement of neurologic symptoms can be seen in up to 70% of patients, as well improvement of quality of life and better outcomes in most of the patients.[3,6,14]

ANKYLOSING SPONDYLITIS

Ankylosing spondylitis (AS) is a chronic inflammatory disease of the sacroiliac joints and spine leading to ankylosis, or severe spinal restriction due to bony or fibrous bridging of the joints. Symptoms commonly begin in late adolescence and early adulthood, with males more commonly affected than females in a 2:1 ratio.[15] The prevalence of AS varies in different populations from 0.1% in some African and Eskimo populations to 0.5% to 1% among white populations in the United Kingdom and the United States.[16] Some feel that the prevalence of AS reflects the prevalence of HLA-B27 in different populations.[17]

Clinical features of this disease include back pain caused by sacroiliitis and inflammation at other locations in the axial skeleton, as well as peripheral arthritis and enthesitis. The most notable feature of this disease is back pain. Back pain associated with AS is an inflammatory back pain, which has different characteristics than mechanical back pain. Symptoms suggestive of inflammatory back pain include onset before the age of 40 years, insidious onset, improvement with exercise, no improvement with rest, and pain at night that improves upon arising.[18] Alternating or asymmetric buttock pain may be indicative of sacroiliac involvement. Groin pain is a relatively common complaint, indicative of arthritis or entheseal disease of the hips. Inflammation at the insertion of the supraspinatus tendon into the greater tuberosity of the humerus may cause shoulder pain and limited mobility. Finally, enthesitis may manifest as tenderness at costochondral junctions, the calcaneal attachments of the Achilles tendon and the plantar fascia, and along the superior iliac crest.

There are no pathognomonic physical findings, but the presence of limited spinal and/or chest mobility are suggestive of AS. Postural abnormalities such as increased flexion of the neck, increased thoracic kyphosis, and loss of normal lumbar lordosis may result from years of disease activity. Specific measurements documenting motion of the back and chest can help assess progression of the disease from baseline and response to treatment. For example, the Schober test can assess lumbar spine mobility. Additionally, measurement of occiput-to-wall distance assesses spinal mobility; increased occiput-to-wall distance is indicative of loss of lumbar and cervical lordosis and increasing thoracic spinal kyphosis. Also, chest wall expansion can be measured at the level of the 4th intercostal space at maximal forced expiration followed by maximal inspiration. Normal expansion is usually considered to be 5 cm or more, with less than 2.5 cm interpreted as abnormal. Other physical examination findings include sacroiliac joint tenderness, flexion deformities of the hip, peripheral joint synovitis, and entheseal tenderness and/or swelling.

Laboratory assessment should include CRP and determination of the presence or absence of HLA-B27. HLA-B27 is most useful in patients with chronic back pain with inflammatory features.[19] Radiographic abnormality is a hallmark of the diagnosis of AS. Squaring of the vertebral bodies due to anterior and posterior spondylitis is an early sign of inflammatory and destructive spinal involvement. Syndesmophytes and ankylosis are the most characteristic features of this disease, which can be visible on conventional radiographs after months to years.[20] Although there are many possible radiographic views of the hips, a simple anteroposterior view of the pelvis allows for assessment of sacroiliac joint changes such as widening, erosions, sclerosis, or ankylosis. However, even after 10 years of disease only 40 percent of AS patients have radiographic evidence of sacroiliitis on plain films.[21] If there are no demonstrable radiographic changes on plain films, but the clinical suspicion for AS is high, then MRI of the pelvis is a much more sensitive imaging modality and can identify sacroiliitis earlier.[22,23] Bone marrow edema is the diagnostic MRI sign of spondylitis.[23] Ultimately, the diagnosis of AS is made from a combination of suggestive clinical features and evidence of sacroiliitis on imaging.

An important issue for nonrheumatologists is that there is a long delay between the occurrence of the first symptoms and the final diagnosis of AS, reported in several studies to be 5 to 10 years or even higher, with longer delays in females.[15,24] Early diagnosis of AS is important because (1) it avoids unnecessary diagnostic procedures and inappropriate treatments; (2) there are effective treatment options including nonsteroidal antiinflammatory drugs (NSAIDs) and tumor necrosis factor (TNF)-blocking agents, with TNF antagonists being very effective in early disease; and (3) patients with early disease but no radiographic sacroiliitis and those with established AS have a similar level of pain and disease activity and, therefore, need an equally aggressive level of treatment.[25] Consequently, some experts suggest that physicians should refer any patient with the clinical symptom of inflammatory back pain or any patient with chronic back pain and a positive HLA-B27 test to a rheumatologist for further evaluation.[19]

In addition to musculoskeletal symptoms, physicians must be aware of extraarticular manifestations such as anterior uveitis, psoriasis, inflammatory bowel disease, or, rarely, aortic root dilatation and conduction abnormalities. Clinical signs such as diarrhea, skin or nail problems, eye discomfort, redness or pain, and unexplained weight loss or fever should alert the physician to the need for further investigation.[26] Unilateral uveitis, presenting with acute pain, photophobia, and blurring of vision, is the most common extra-articular complication of AS, occurring in about 33.2% of patients.[27] Ileocolonoscopic evidence of gut inflammation is present in up to 60% of AS patients, unrelated to gastrointestinal complaints, with a fraction of these patients evolving into true inflammatory bowel disease over time.[26] Constitutionally, patients may also experience significant fatigue. Of note, not only is this disease specifically associated with aortic valve disease and conduction disturbances, but patients with AS have a higher risk of cardiovascular disease as well.

Important risks associated with AS include fracture of the ankylosed spine and atlantoaxial subluxation, which can lead to unusual neck and back pain. AS patients with persistently active disease often have decreased bone mineral density leading to osteopenia or osteoporosis.[28] Patients with ankylosed spines can develop fractures with minimal trauma such as riding a truck over rough terrain, and sometimes with even no recollected trauma.[29] Additionally, there are multiple case reports in the literature as well as a study of Mexican patients that highlight the risk of cervical subluxation due to ligamentous calcification and cervical ossification.[30–32] Consequently, the possibility of spinal fracture or atlantoaxial subluxation must be considered whenever a patient with AS develops unusual neck or back pain. Patients with unrecognized fractures can commonly complain of axial pain until abrupt neurologic deterioration occurs. Therefore, because of difficulties in radiographically visualizing the spine in AS, screening of the entire spinal column with advanced neuroimaging with MRI or CT scan is recommended.[33,34]

Exercise or physiotherapy and NSAIDs have traditionally formed the cornerstone of treatment for AS.[35] There has been no evidence supporting the use DMARDs, including sulfasalazine and methotrexate, for the treatment of axial disease, although sulfasalazine may be considered in patients with peripheral arthritis.[36] More recently, biologic agents have contributed significantly to the management of AS. TNF treatment should be considered in patients with persistently high disease activity despite conventional therapy.[36] Based on current data, among TNF inhibitors, the monoclonal antibodies infliximab and adalimumab, are more appropriate than etanercept if extra-articular manifestations or comorbid conditions, such as uveitis or inflammatory bowel disease, are present or suspected.[26] In the end, the treatment of AS should be tailored according to the manifestations of the disease at presentation, severity of symptoms, as well as the wishes and expectations of the patient.[20]

DERMATOMYOSITIS AND POLYMYOSITIS

Dermatomyositis (DM) and polymyositis (PM) are inflammatory myopathies characterized by muscle weakness and frequently elevated levels of serum muscle enzymes. Both disorders have an estimated prevalence of about 1 per 100,000, with a female to male predominance of about 2 to 1. Although individuals of all ages can be affected, peak incidence occurs between the ages of 40 and 50 years.[37] Histopathologically, these two diseases share the findings of muscle fiber necrosis, degeneration, regeneration, and inflammatory cell infiltrate.[38]

DM and PM can present with a wide range of clinical symptoms, the most prominent of which is muscle weakness and low muscle endurance. The onset of muscle weakness is usually insidious, with a gradual worsening over several months. The distribution of weakness is typically symmetric and proximal, rather than distal.[39] Specifically, many of the muscles of the trunk, shoulders, hips, upper arms, and thighs are usually involved.[40] Notably, the pharyngeal and neck extensor muscles are often involved, causing dysphagia and difficulty in holding up the head. In restricted forms of the disease, only the neck or paraspinal muscles are affected.[41] Patients generally report difficulty walking uphill or upstairs, brushing or washing their hair, or rising from chairs. Although distal muscle weakness can occur, it is usually mild and does not cause significant functional impairment. Additionally, myalgias and muscle tenderness can occur in up to 50 percent of cases, but these muscle pains are typically milder than that of patients with polymyalgia rheumatica, fibromyalgia, and viral or bacterial myositis.

Clinically, the presence of several distinct skin rashes differentiates DM from PM. A raised violaceous or erythematous scaly eruption may occur symmetrically over the metacarpophalangeal and interphalangeal joints, known as Gottron papules. Similar lesions can also be seen over the extensor aspects of the elbows and knees, mimicking psoriasis. Patients also commonly present with a heliotrope rash, a red-purple eruption on the upper eyelids, often accompanied with periorbital edema. The shawl sign may be present, in which patients are noted to have a diffuse, flat erythematous lesion over the chest and shoulders in the distribution of a shawl. A similar rash, when present in a V-shaped distribution over the anterior neck and chest, is the V-sign. These rashes are exacerbated by sun exposure. Patients with active disease can have widespread erythema, called erythroderma, over the trunk and extremities. Patients with DM often have skin lesions on their fingers, such as peri-ungual erythema, nail-fold telangiectasias, and cuticular overgrowth. Finally, a dermatologic finding shared by patients with both DM and PM is mechanic's hands. Patients can be found to have hyperkeratosis, or thickened, rough, and cracked skin at the tips and lateral aspects of the fingers as well as of the palms.[42,43]

A more significant clinical manifestation of DM and PM, in that it is a major risk factor for morbidity and mortality, is lung involvement. Patients may experience cough or dyspnea, related to either weakness of the respiratory muscles or interstitial lung disease. Interstitial lung disease, caused by inflammation in the small airways, is often associated with antisynthetase autoantibodies.[44,45] The severity of interstitial lung disease may vary from mild or asymptomatic to rapidly progressive.

Another clinical manifestation of PM and DM is cardiac involvement. Patients may have conduction abnormalities and arrhythmias related to myocarditis and coronary artery disease, as well as involvement of the small vessels of the myocardium. Thus, examination with ECG and assessment of the serum troponins is recommended in newly diagnosed patients with PM or DM.[46] Commonly, patients may have joint pain and arthritis. This arthritis is typically a symmetric, nonerosive arthritis of the small joints of the hands and feet.

Diagnosis of DM and PM is made from observation of the aforementioned clinical findings in the context of elevated serum muscle enzymes and autoantibodies. It is important to rule out other causes of muscle weakness and muscle damage such as neurologic or metabolic disorders, HIV, use of prescription or illicit drugs, or other connective tissue diseases.

Most patients with DM or PM have elevations of muscle enzymes including creatinine kinase, lactate dehydrogenase, aldolase, aspartate aminotransferase, and alanine aminotransferase at some point during the course of the disease. There is a correlation between the severity of weakness and level of enzyme elevation,[37] but the degree of muscle dysfunction may be greater than the level of muscle enzyme abnormalities suggest. Antinuclear antibody (ANA) testing is frequently positive in patients with DM and PM. Specific autoantibody testing such as anti-Sm, SS-A, SS-B, and antiribonucleoprotein, can be useful for diagnosis of connective tissue disorders associated with myositis such as lupus. Other, more myositis-specific, autoantibodies such as anti-Jo-1, antibodies to signal recognition particles, and antibodies to Mi-2, can indicate prognosis and future patterns of organ involvement. Specifically, anti-Jo-1 antibodies are associated with interstitial lung disease, Raynaud phenomenon, mechanic's hands, and arthritis, the antisynthetase phenomenon.[45]

Additional testing, including skin biopsy, electromyography, muscle biopsy, or MRI, may be ordered in patients in whom other tests are inconclusive. Notably, an association between DM-PM and malignancy has been observed.[47,48] As such, it is imperative to screen for malignancy in patients at the time of diagnosis and at relapse, particularly if the symptoms do not respond to conventional immunosuppressive treatment.[49] Screening for malignancies should include a careful clinical examination, routine blood tests, chest radiograph, along with any other age-appropriate screenings.

Determinants of prognosis in DM and PM include time to diagnosis, amount of weakness at presentation, autoantibody profile, and the presence of extramuscular disease features such as interstitial lung disease or dysphagia. Irrespective of prognosis, the goals of therapy are to improve muscle strength and to avoid development of extramuscular complications. The mainstay of therapy for DM and PM is the use of systemic corticosteroids. Traditionally, prednisone is given at a dose of 1 mg/kg daily as initial therapy for several months to establish control of disease. Steroids should then be tapered slowly to the lowest effective dose with a total duration of therapy around 9 to 12 months. Early intervention with a steroid-sparing immunosuppressive agent such as methotrexate or azathioprine should be initiated to induce or maintain remission. Other immunosuppressive agents can be used such as chlorambucil, cyclosporine, cyclophosphamide, mycophenolate mofetil, rituximab, TNF antagonists, and high-dose intravenous immune globulin, especially when confronted with resistant disease.[50] As previously mentioned, in the face of resistant disease, it is important to investigate for an unrecognized malignancy.

DIFFUSE IDIOPATHIC SKELETAL HYPEROSTOSIS

Diffuse idiopathic skeletal hyperostosis (DISH), also known as Forestier disease and ankylosing hyperostosis, is a noninflammatory condition characterized by calcification and ossification of spinal ligaments and entheses, where tendons and ligaments attach to bone. The incidence varies by population and increases with age, such that DISH is rarely diagnosed before the age of 40. It has also been noted that there is a male predominance of the disease.[51] At this time, the cause and pathogenesis of DISH remains unknown. However, it is seen more commonly in patients with metabolic disorders such as obesity, hypertension, glucose intolerance or overt diabetes, hyperuricemia, and the metabolic syndrome.[52,53] Interestingly, mechanical factors may play a role. Bony bridging is usually more prominent on the right side of the thoracic spine in patients with DISH; whereas, in patients with DISH and dextrocardia or situs inversus, there is more extensive bony bridging on the left side of the thoracic spine.[54]

Symptoms of DISH vary from mild back pain and/or slight loss of function to severe complications such as dysphagia, myelopathy, and spinal canal stenosis. Most frequently, patients report pain in the thoracic spine, but patients with DISH can have neck, low back, and/or extremity pain. Although this condition in not known to be inflammatory, about 80% of patients experience spinal morning stiffness.[55] Cervical involvement can cause hoarseness, stridor, aspiration pneumonia, sleep apnea, atlantoaxial subluxation, thoracic outlet syndrome, or most commonly dysphagia caused by compression of the esophagus by large anterior cervical osteophytes.[56] More deleterious, involvement of the posterior longitudinal ligament of the cervical spine can result in spinal cord compression and myelopathy.

The most common physical examination finding is decreased range of spinal motion, particularly loss of thoracic lateral flexion. Often patients are found to have tenderness over entheses or even palpable nodules at the entheses, most commonly at the elbow, knee, and Achilles region. Patients may have palpable bony spurs of the calcaneus, olecranon, and patella. These physical findings, in conjunction with a history of recurrent Achilles tendonitis, recurrent shoulder "bursitis," recurrent lateral or medial epicondylitis, dysphagia, or myelopathy are important clinical clues in the diagnosis of DISH.[55]

The diagnostic hallmarks of DISH are radiographic abnormalities. DISH is characterized by the ossification of paravertebral ligaments and peripheral entheses. Flowing linear calcification and ossification can be seen along the anterolateral aspects of the vertebral bodies, which continues across the disc space. These findings are more prominent on the right side of the thoracic spine. At times, ossification of the posterior longitudinal ligament of the cervical spine may also be present.[55,57–59]

Because this condition is more prevalent in older individuals, DISH and osteoarthritis often coexist. However, radiographic findings present in degenerative disc disease, including marginal sclerosis of vertebral bodies, disc calcification, or the vacuum phenomena, are rare in any spinal region in DISH.[54,57,58] If the diagnosis of DISH is suspected, then radiographic evaluation of the spine, particularly the thoracic spine, should be performed. Previous chest radiographs should also be reviewed if available.

A number of conditions can produce spinal bony abnormalities similar to those observed in DISH, including spondylosis deformans, ankylosing spondylitis, acromegaly, hypoparathyroidism, fluorosis, trauma, retinoid use, ochronosis, and X-linked hypophosphatemic osteomalacia. Of the conditions listed, spondylosis deformans and AS are the most frequently considered in the differential diagnosis of DISH. Radiographically, both DISH and AS manifest as ligamentous ossification and syndesmophytes. In ankylosing spondylitis, the syndesmophytes are slender, vertical bony bridges that involve the outer margin of the annulus fibrosis, as compared with involvement of the anterior longitudinal ligament in DISH. Furthermore, in DISH there are classically no erosions or bony ankylosis of the sacroiliac and apophyseal joints, which is characteristic of ankylosing spondylitis. In regard to spondylosis deformans, spurs seen in the cervical and lumbar spine can resemble those seen in DISH. However, involvement of the anterior longitudinal ligament in the thoracic spine, a distinguishing feature of DISH, is not seen in spondylosis.[57,60]

There is no specific treatment that can halt the process of DISH. A high degree of bony bridging is associated with a lower pain threshold and, consequently, with a lower functional status.[61] Treatment is targeted toward symptoms, specifically pain relief and maintaining physical function. Mild pain can often be treated with acetaminophen or NSAIDs. Physical function can be maintained and improved with range of motion and stretching exercises, as well as with exercise programs.[62] Surgical intervention is occasionally required to treat dysphagia caused by large cervical spurs, or more significantly, to intervene in a situation of progressive myelopathy caused by ossification of the posterior longitudinal ligament of the cervical spine.

Special considerations in patients with DISH include potential complexity in airway management due to intubation difficulty and the risk of spinal cord injury.[63] It is also important to note that, because patients with DISH may have a long history of back pain and because interpretation of their radiographs can be difficult due to pathologic osseous changes, they have an increased risk of delayed fracture diagnosis.[64]

POLYMYALGIA RHEUMATICA AND GIANT CELL ARTERITIS

Polymyalgia rheumatica (PMR) and giant cell arteritis (GCA) are closely related conditions that affect persons of middle age and older, and frequently occur together.

Controversy remains as to whether PMR and GCA are the same disease or whether they are two different but often concurrent conditions.[65,66] The incidence of PMR and GCA increases after the age of 50 years and peaks between 70 and 80 years of age. Due to the progressive aging of the population in Western countries, both conditions have emerged as relatively common diseases in the elderly.[67]

GCA, also known as temporal arteritis, is the most common systemic vasculitis in adults. GCA affects medium-sized and large-sized arteries.[68] The most commonly affected populations include Scandinavians and northern Europeans greater than 50 years of age, with a female gender predominance.[69] Overall, the incidence of GCA is 15 to 25 per 100,000 per year in individuals more than 50 years old.

GCA has a wide spectrum of clinical manifestations related to both systemic inflammation and ischemia. It was first described by Fay,[70] in 1927, as a neck pain syndrome and later defined by the International Headache Society,[71,72] in 1988, as a distinct entity with pain involving the affected side of the neck, possibly projecting to the same side of the head. It is now known that the most common presenting clinical signs are headache, scalp tenderness, jaw claudication, acute visual disturbances such as blurring or diplopia, and constitutional symptoms, including fever, weight loss, anorexia, and malaise. Of note, the most common symptom is headache, while the most specific is jaw claudication.[73,74] On examination, patients may have a tender or thickened superficial temporal artery with reduced or absent pulsation, upper cranial nerve palsies, or if large-vessel GCA is present, then vascular bruits and asymmetry of pulses or blood pressure may be elicited.[73]

There is no pathognomonic laboratory test for the diagnosis of GCA. Specific autoantibodies have not been identified. Patients often have abnormal laboratory findings indicating an acute-phase response such as a high erythrocyte sedimentation rate (ESR) (often 100 mm/h or more), an elevated CRP, normocytic anemia, thrombocytosis, low albumin, and abnormal liver function tests such as an elevated alkaline phosphatase.[75] Treatment decisions, however, should not be predicated on laboratory results as an elevated acute phase response may not be present in all patients.[76–78]

Diagnosis of GCA is made from a combined assessment of clinical findings, laboratory tests, and histopathology. The role of imaging modalities such as MRI or angiography, conventional angiography, Doppler ultrasound, and positron emission tomography requires further investigation before their clinical utility can be defined. If a patient more than 50 years of age presents with the features discussed above, the diagnosis of GCA should be considered. Corticosteroid treatment should be started immediately, followed by temporal artery biopsy. Prompt initiation of corticosteroid therapy and close follow-up of these patients is warranted to minimize the risk of irreversible vision loss.

Temporal artery biopsy is the gold standard for diagnosis, revealing inflammatory cell infiltration of arterial walls with or without giant cells and disruption of the internal elastic lamina leading to luminal occlusion and tissue ischemia.[69] These lesions are focal and segmental with "skip lesions." Thus, histologic signs of inflammation may be missed in temporal artery biopsy performed in arteritis-free segments.[79] Nonetheless, steroid therapy should not be withheld pending temporal artery biopsy as histopathological findings persist even after more than 14 days after steroid initiation.[80] Steroids should be initiated at 1 mg/kg for a minimum of 4 weeks, after which time they should be tapered on the basis of symptoms and serial monitoring of inflammatory markers. There is inadequate data to recommend the initiation of a cytotoxic agent such as methotrexate, azathioprine, cyclophosphamide, dapsone, cyclosporine, or TNF antagonists as steroid-sparing therapy.[81,82] Aspirin, however, may be an important adjunctive treatment as retrospective studies have shown reductions in the risks of visual loss and central nervous system ischemic events among patients taking aspirin for other reasons at the time that GCA was diagnosed.[83,84]

PMR is a closely related systemic inflammatory disease that may occur on a spectrum in the same population as GCA.[68] PMR occurs two to three times more frequently,[75] and may present as an isolated entity or be seen in patients who later develop typical cranial manifestations of GCA.

PMR is a syndrome characterized by aching and morning stiffness in the neck, shoulder, and/or pelvic girdles in persons 50 years or older for at least 4 weeks. Patients most often complain of relatively acute onset of aching and pain in the muscles of the neck, shoulders, low back, hips, thighs, and occasionally the trunk with resultant difficulties in rising and dressing. Such myalgias are often accompanied by systemic manifestations including low-grade fever, fatigue, and weight loss. Patients may also experience morning stiffness that typically lasts at least 30 minutes.[75,85]

On examination, active, and often passive, range of motion of the neck, shoulders, and hips is limited due to pain. The shoulders may even be tender to palpation. Distal musculoskeletal manifestations are seen in about half of patients including mild to moderate synovitis, often in the wrists and knees, carpal tunnel syndrome, and distal extremity swelling of the dorsum of the hands and wrists, ankles, and dorsum of the feet.[85] Subdeltoid and subacromial bursitis or, less commonly, glenohumeral or biceps tendonitis, may be found due to inflammation of the periarticular structures.[75] Notably, muscle strength is usually normal, although patients may complain of weakness.

Unlike GCA, there is no gold standard test for the diagnosis of PMR, and other conditions may mimic or share polymyalgic features such as malignancy and seronegative polyarthritis.[86] Most patients have increased acute phase reactants including high ESR and CRP levels, and anemia of chronic disease. Serologic tests, such as antinuclear antibodies, rheumatoid factor, and cyclic citrullinated peptide antibodies, are typically negative.[85,87] Imaging with MRI or ultrasonography can detect underlying inflammation of a bursitis or tenosynovitis,[88,89] but is not needed for diagnosis.

Although temporal artery biopsy can be deferred in patients with PMR in whom no signs of GCA are present,[90] these patients must be followed closely because a small proportion of such patients have or develop GCA within several months despite receiving steroid treatment for PMR.[91]

PMR remission, when not associated with GCA, can be achieved with prednisone treatment at a dose of 15 mg/day in most patients. Reductions below 10 mg/day of prednisone should preferably follow a tapering rate of less than 1 mg/month such that patients receive steroid therapy for at least a year. No medication has been consistently proven as a steroid sparing agent. To reduce the total cumulative dose of glucocorticoids and their adverse effects, methotrexate has often been suggested.[92] Small pilot studies have advocated the use of TNF antagonists such as etanercept and infliximab,[93–95] but efficacy has not been demonstrated in at least one randomized-controlled trial.[96]

FIBROMYALGIA SYNDROME

Fibromyalgia syndrome is a diffuse pain syndrome of unknown cause associated with the presence on physical examination of multiple tender points.[97] This is a common rheumatic disorder affecting 1% to 4% of the population; about 75% of these patients are female.[98]

Fibromyalgia is characterized by generalized musculoskeletal pain; the patient describes pain "all over," bilaterally, involving upper and lower extremities. In initial stages of the disease, pain can be localized in the neck and shoulder muscles. Often pain is associated with other symptoms such as fatigue, paresthesias, weakness,[99] joint swelling, cognitive disturbances, insomnia, sleep disorders,[100] and symptoms suggestive of irritable bowel syndrome.[101,102] The physical examination is usually unremarkable except for the presence of tenderness in specific locations. Diagnosis requires the presence of pain on palpation of 11 of the 18 established tender points when pressure is applied at 4 kg/cm^2.[97]

Although the presence of multiple nonspecific symptoms can be observed in many conditions, the history and physical examination are usually helpful in differentiating fibromyalgia from other pain syndromes. Routine laboratory testing, including complete blood cell count, ESR, and CRP, is normal, as are imaging studies. In patients with symptoms suggestive of thyroid disease, muscle disease, or inflammatory rheumatic disease, appropriate testing including serum creatine kinase, thyroid function tests, and ANA would be useful if a high clinical suspicion exists. Additional evaluation with sleep studies in patients with insomnia or referral to mental health for mood disorders should be considered.

Fibromyalgia is not uncommon in patients with other rheumatic conditions such as RA, systemic lupus erythematosus, Sjögren syndrome, AS, and polymyalgia rheumatica.[97,98] Distinction between fibromyalgia pain and disease activity is important when making decisions regarding further treatment.[103]

The variety of symptoms and syndromes that can coexist with this diagnosis include tension or migraine headaches, irritable bowel syndrome,[101,104] irritable bladder, chronic fatigue syndrome, vulvodynia, temporomandibular dysfunction, nondermatomal paresthesias, multiple chemical sensitivities, and noncardiac chest pain or dyspnea.[105,106] Osteoarthritis, muscle strains, and spinal stenosis may be present or mimic fibromyalgia but these disorders are associated with localized rather that widespread pain.

The treatment of fibromyalgia involves education, exercise, cognitive behavioral therapy, stress management, sleep improvement, and pharmacologic therapy. Education about the nature and benign nonprogressive course of the condition is critical, as well the importance of a multidisciplinary approach.[107,108] NSAIDs have been shown not to be particularly effective, although tramadol in combination with acetaminophen has some modest results.[109] There is no evidence supporting the use of narcotics for this condition. Psychotropic agents such as tricyclic antidepressants, serotonin reuptake inhibitors, and norepinephrine-serotonin reuptake inhibitors have shown to be effective in the treatment of fibromyalgia.[110,111] Anticonvulsivants such as gabapentin,[112] pregabalin,[110,113–115] and clonazepam have been shown to decrease pain and have the additional benefit of aiding with sleep.

Outcomes improve when aerobic exercise is added to the regimen. Low-impact routines such as swimming,[116] walking, and biking are recommended. Patients should be recommended to start low and go slow to reduce any aches and pains associated with exercises and improve adherence to a long-term exercise regimen.[117,118] Cognitive behavioral therapy teaches skills directed to reduce pain such as relaxation techniques, distraction, and pleasant activities scheduling.[119] Other areas that should be considered include sleep hygiene, management of anxiety and/or depression, and goal setting. Other modalities used for symptom management include tai chi, chiropractic manipulations, massage therapy, acupuncture,[120] and trigger point injections.[107] Further review of complementary treatments is covered elsewhere in this issue.

Myofascial pain syndrome overlaps considerably with fibromyalgia. Patients with myofascial pain syndrome complain of pain in one anatomic region, with pain localized to that area. Many of the original reports of fibromyalgia actually described what would now be termed myofascial pain syndrome. Some of the confusion lies in the differentiation between trigger points and tender points.[121] Myofascial pain is defined by the presence of trigger points that are found in a taut band in the muscle with a characteristic referred pain when pressure is applied to the trigger point.[122] Fibromyalgia tender points are soft tissue sites that are excessively tender on palpation. Within the myofascial pain syndromes are other pain disorders such as tension headaches,[123] cervical strain disorders, and work-related musculoskeletal disorder. The presence of pain is often associated with neurovestibular abnormalities such as dizziness and neurocognitive disturbances. Myofascial pain may respond well to local treatment.[108] Modalities such as cold spray, passive stretch of the involved muscle, and trigger point injections have shown some effectiveness in clinical trials.[124–128] The response to treatment on myofascial pain is generally better then that of fibromyalgia.[122,129,130]

SUMMARY

Many different rheumatic conditions can present with cervicalgia. Musculoskeletal neck pain is a symptom in the vast majority of rheumatic diseases. Other considerations include infections, which are more common in patients who may be on immunosuppressive therapy for their underlying illness. In addition, rheumatology patients are not exempt from common sports injuries, and these diagnoses should be considered. Further discussion about sports injuries and neck pain is reviewed elsewhere in this issue. With the appropriate diagnostic work up, a systemic inflammatory illness can be detected in a timely fashion and the appropriate therapy can be instituted to avoid progression and complications.

REFERENCES

1. Krauss WE, Bledsoe JM, Clarke MJ, et al. Rheumatoid arthritis of the craniovertebral junction. Neurosurgery 2010;66(Suppl 3):83–95.
2. Kim DH, Hilibrand AS. Rheumatoid arthritis in the cervical spine. J Am Acad Orthop Surg 2005;13:463–74.
3. Wolfs FC, Kloppenburg M, Fehlings MG, et al. Neurologic outcome of surgical and conservative treatment of rheumatoid cervical spine subluxation: a systematic review. Arthritis Rheum 2009;61:1743–52.
4. Narvaez JA, Narvaez J, de Albert M, et al. Bone marrow edema in the cervical spine of symptomatic rheumatoid arthritis patients. Semin Arthritis Rheum 2009; 38:281–8.
5. Nguyen HV, Ludwing SC, Solber JK, et al. Rheumatoid arthritis of the cervical spine. Spine J 2004;4(3):329–34.
6. Neo M. Treatment of upper cervical spine involvement in rheumatoid arthritis patients. Mod Rheumatol 2008;18:327–35.
7. Neva MH, Hakkinen A, Makinen H, et al. High prevalence of asymptomatic cervical spine subluxation in patients with rheumatoid arthritis waiting for orthopaedic surgery. Ann Rheum Dis 2006;65:884–8.
8. Hamilton JD, Johnston RA, Madhok R, et al. Factors predictive of subsequent deterioration in rheumatoid cervical myelopathy. Rheumatology (Oxford) 2001; 40:811–5.
9. Neva MH, Kauppi MJ, Kautiainen H, et al. Combination drug therapy retards the development of rheumatoid atlantoaxial subluxations. FIN-RACo Trial Group. Arthritis Rheum 2000;43:2397–401.

10. Kauppi MJ, Neva MH, Laiho K, et al. Rheumatoid atlantoaxial subluxation can be prevented by intensive use of traditional disease modifying antirheumatic drugs. J Rheumatol 2009;36:273.
11. Hakkinen A, Makinen H, Ylinen J, et al. Stability of the upper neck during isometric neck exercises in rheumatoid arthritis patients with atlantoaxial disorders. Scand J Rheumatol 2008;37(5):343–7.
12. Schmitt-Sody M, Kirchhoff C, Buhmann S, et al. Timing of cervical spine stabilization and outcome in patients with rheumatoid arthritis. Int Orthop 2008;32:511–6.
13. Matsunaga S, Sakou T, Onishi T, et al. Prognosis of patients with upper cervical lesions caused by rheumatoid arthritis: comparison of occipitocervical fusion between C1 laminectomy and nonsurgical management. Spine 2003;28:1581–7.
14. Paus AC, Steen H, Roislien J, et al. High mortality rate in rheumatoid arthritis with subluxation of the cervical spine: a cohort study of operated and nonoperated patients. Spine (Phila Pa 1976) 2008;33:2278–83.
15. Feldtkeller E, Khan MA, van der Heijde D, et al. Age at disease onset and diagnosis delay in HLAB27 negative vs. positive patients with ankylosing spondylitis. Rheumatol Int 2003;23(2):61–6.
16. Klippel JH. Seronegative spondyloarthropathies, Ankylosing spondylitis. In: Primer on the Rheumatic Diseases. 12th edition. Georgia (Atlanta): Arthritis Foundation; 2001. p. 250–5.
17. Khan MA. Epidemiology of HLA-B27 and arthritis. Clin Rheumatol 1996;15:10–2.
18. Sieper J, van der Heijde D, Landewe R, et al. New criteria for inflammatory back pain in patients with chronic back pain: a real patient exercise by experts from the Assessment of SpondyloArthritis International Society (ASAS). Ann Rheum Dis 2009;68:784–8.
19. Rudwaleit M, van der Heijde D, Khan MA, et al. How to diagnose axial spondyloarthritis early. Ann Rheum Dis 2004;63:535–43.
20. Braun J, Sieper J. Ankylosing spondylitis. Lancet 2007;369:1379–90.
21. Huerta-Sil G, Casasola-Vargas JC, Londona JD, et al. Low grade radiographic sacroiliitis as prognostic factor in patients with undifferentiated spondyloarthritis fulfilling diagnostic criteria for ankylosing spondylitis throughout follow up. Ann Rheum Dis 2006;65(5):642–6.
22. Oostveen J, Prevo R, den Boer J, et al. Early detection of sacroiliitis on magnetic resonance imaging and subsequent development of sacroiliitis on plain radiography. A prospective, longitudinal study. J Rheumatol 1999;26:1953–8.
23. Maksymowych WP, Landewe R. Imaging in ankylosing spondylitis. Best Pract Res Clin Rheumatol 2006;20(3):507–19.
24. Calin A, Elswood J, Rigg S, et al. Ankylosing spondylitis—an analytical review of 1500 patients: the changing pattern of disease. J Rheumatol 1988;15(8):1234–8.
25. Song IH, Sieper J, Rudwaleit M. Diagnosing early ankylosing spondylitis. Curr Rheumatol Rep 2007;9:367–74.
26. Elewaut D, Matucci-Cerinic M. Treatment of ankylosing spondylitis and extra-articular manifestations in everyday rheumatology practice. Rheumatology (Oxford) 2009;48(9):1029–35.
27. Zeboulon N, Dougados M, Gossec L. Prevalence and characteristics of uveitis in the spondyloarthropathies: a systematic literature review. Ann Rheum Dis 2008;67(7):955–9.
28. Dos Santos FP, Constantin A, Laroche M, et al. Whole body and regional bone mineral density in ankylosing spondylitis. J Rheumatol 2001;28(3):547–9.

29. Smith MD, Scott JM, Murali R, et al. Minor neck trauma in chronic ankylosing spondylitis: a potentially fatal combination. J Clin Rheumatol 2007;13(2):81–4.
30. Toussirot E, Benmansour A, Bonneville JF, et al. Atlantoaxial subluxation in an ankylosing spondylitis patient with cervical spine ossification. Br J Rheumatol 1997;36(2):293–5.
31. Chen WS, Lee HT, Tsai CY, et al. Severe atlantoaxial subluxation in early ankylosing spondylitis. J Clin Rheumatol 2010;16(7):353.
32. Ramos-Remus C, Gomez-Vargas A, Guzman-Guzman JL, et al. Frequency of atlantoaxial subluxation and neurologic involvement in patients with ankylosing spondylitis. J Rheumatol 1995;22(11):2120–5.
33. Finkelstein J, Chapman JR, Mirza S. Occult vertebral fractures in Ankylosing spondylitis. Spinal Cord 1999;376:444–7.
34. Caron T, Bransford R, Nguyen Q, et al. Spine fractures in patients with Ankylosing spinal disorders. Spine 2010;35:58–64.
35. Dougados M, Dijkmans B, Khan M, et al. Conventional treatment for Ankylosing spondylitis. Ann Rheum Dis 2002;61:40–50.
36. Zochling J, van der Heijde D, Burgos-Vargas R, et al. ASAS/EULAR recommendations for the management of ankylosing spondylitis. Ann Rheum Dis 2006; 65(4):442–52.
37. Tymms KE, Webb J. Dermatomyositis and other connective tissue diseases: a review of 105 cases. J Rheumatol 1985;12:1140–8.
38. Dalakas MC. Muscle biopsy findings in inflammatory myopathies. Rheum Dis Clin North Am 2002;28:779–98.
39. Hochberg MC, Feldman D, Stevens MB. Adult onset polymyositis/dermatomyositis: an analysis of clinical and laboratory features and survival in 76 patients with a review of the literature. Semin Arthritis Rheum 1986;15(3):168–78.
40. Harris-Love MO, Shrader JA, Koziol D, et al. Distribution and severity of weakness among patients with polymyositis, dermatomyositis and juvenile dermatomyositis. Rheumatology (Oxford) 2009;48(2):134–9.
41. Kuo SH, Vullaganti M, Jimenez-Shahed J, et al. Camptocormia as a presentation of generalized inflammatory myopathy. Muscle Nerve 2009;40:1059–63.
42. Sunkureddi P, Nguyen-Oghalai T, Jarvis J, et al. Clinical signs of dermatomyositis. Hosp Physician 2005;41(3):41–4.
43. Callen JP, Wortmann RL. Dermatomyositis. Clin Dermatol 2006;24:363–73.
44. Marie I, Hatron P-Y, Hachulla E, et al. Pulmonary involvement in polymyositis and in dermatomyositis. J Rheumatol 1998;25:1336–43.
45. Fathi M, Dastmalchi M, Rasmussen E, et al. Interstitial lung disease, a common manifestation of newly diagnosed polymyositis and dermatomyositis. Ann Rheum Dis 2004;63:297–301.
46. Gonzalez-Lopez L, Gamez-Nava JI, Sanchez L, et al. Cardiac manifestations in dermato-polymyositis. Clin Exp Rheumatol 1996;14:373–9.
47. Airio A, Pukkala E, Isomäki H. Elevated cancer incidence in patients with dermatomyositis: a population based study. J Rheumatol 1995;22:1300–3.
48. Sigurgeirsson B, Lindelöf B, Edhag O, et al. Risk of cancer in patients with dermatomyositis or polymyositis. N Engl J Med 1992;325:363–7.
49. Buchbinder R, Hill CL. Malignancy in patients with inflammatory myopathy. Curr Rheumatol Rep 2002;4(5):415–26.
50. Choy EH, Isenberg DA. Treatment of dermatomyositis and polymyositis. Rheumatology 2002;41:7–13.
51. Belanger TA, Rowe DE. Diffuse idiopathic skeletal hyperostosis: musculoskeletal manifestations. J Am Acad Orthop Surg 2001;9:258–67.

52. Denko CW, Malemud CJ. Body mass index and blood glucose: correlations with serum insulin, growth hormone, and insulin-like growth factor-1 levels in patients with diffuse idiopathic skeletal hyperostosis (DISH). Rheumatol Int 2006;26: 292–7.

53. Kiss C, Szilagyi M, Paksy A, et al. Risk factors for diffuse idiopathic skeletal hyperostosis: a case-control study. Rheumatology (Oxford) 2002;41:27–30.

54. Forestire J, Lagier R. Ankylosing hyperostosis of the spine. Clin Orthop 1971;74: 65–6.

55. Utsinger PD. Diffuse idiopathic skeletal hyperostosis. Clin Rheum Dis 1985;11: 325–6.

56. Mader R. Clinical manifestations of diffuse idiopathic skeletal hyperostosis of the cervical spine. Semin Arthritis Rheum 2002;32:130–2.

57. Resnick D, Niwayama G. Radiographic and pathologic features of spinal involvement in diffuse idiopathic skeletal hyperostosis (DISH). Radiology 1976;119:559–60.

58. Harris J, Carter AR, Glick EN, et al. Ankylosing hyperostosis. I. Clinical and radiological features. Ann Rheum Dis 1974;33:210–1.

59. Fornasier VL, Littlejohn G, Urowitz MB, et al. Spinal entheseal new bone formation: the early changes of spinal diffuse idiopathic skeletal hyperostosis. J Rheumatol 1983;10:939–40.

60. Utsinger PD, Resnick D, Shapiro R. Diffuse skeletal abnormalities in Forestier disease. Arch Intern Med 1976;136:763–4.

61. Mader R, Novofastovski I, Rosner E, et al. Nonarticular tenderness and functional status in patients with Diffuse idiopathic skeletal hyperostosis. J Rheumatol 2010;37:9.

62. Al-Herz A, Snip JP, Clark B, et al. Exercise therapy for patients with diffuse idiopathic skeletal hyperostosis. Clin Rheumatol 2008;27(2):207–10.

63. Ozkalkanli MY, Katircioglu K, Ozkalkanli DT, et al. Airway management of a patient with Forestier's disease. J Anesth 2006;20(4):304–6.

64. Hendrix RW, Melany M, Miller F, et al. Fracture of the spine in patients with ankylosis due to diffuse skeletal hyperostosis: clinical and imaging findings. Am J Roentgenol 1994;162:899–904.

65. Gonzalez-Gay MA. Giant cell arteritis and polymyalgia rheumatica: two different but often overlapping conditions. Semin Arthritis Rheum 2004;33:289–93.

66. Salvarani C, Cantini F, Hunder GG. Polymyalgia rheumatica and giant cell arteritis. Lancet 2008;372:234–45.

67. Gonzalez-Gay MA, Vazquez-Rodriguez TR, Lopez-Diaz MJ, et al. Epidemiology of giant cell arteritis and polymyalgia rheumatica. Arthritis Rheum 2009;61: 1454–61.

68. Chew SSL, Kerr NM, Danesh-Meyer HV. Giant cell arteritis. J Clin Neurosci 2009; 16:1263–8.

69. Wang X, Hu ZP, Lu W, et al. Giant cell arteritis. Rheumatol Int 2008;29(1):1–7.

70. Fay T. Atypical neuralgia. Arch Neurol Psychiat 1927;18:309–15.

71. Headache Classification Committee of the International Headache Society. Classification and diagnoses criteria for headache disorders, cranial neuralgias and facial pain. Cephalalgia 1988;8:48–9.

72. Holland NW, Patel BB. A pain in the neck. Am J Med 2010;123(6):508–9.

73. Kale N, Eggenberger E. Diagnosis and management of giant cell arteritis: a review. Curr Opin Ophthalmol 2010;21:417–22.

74. Smetana GW, Shmerling RH. Does this patient have temporal arteritis? JAMA 2002;2871:92–101.

75. Salvarani C, Cantini S, Boiardi L, et al. Polymyalgia rheumatica and giant cell arteritis. N Engl J Med 2002;347:261–72.
76. Martinez-Taboada VM, Blanco R, Armona J, et al. Giant cell arteritis with an erythrocyte sedimentation rate lower than 50. Clin Rheumatol 2000;19:73–5.
77. Liozon E, Jauberteau-Marchan MO, Ly K, et al. Giant cell arteritis with a low erythrocyte sedimentation rate: comments on the article by Salvarani and Hunder. Arthritis Rheum 2002;47:693–4.
78. Ciccarelli M, Jeanmonod D, Jeanmonod R. Giant cell temporal arteritis with a normal erythrocyte sedimentation rate: report of a case. Am J Emerg Med 2009;27(2):255 e1–3.
79. Klein RG, Campbell RJ, Hunder GG, et al. Skip lesions in temporal arteritis. Mayo Clin Proc 1976;51(8):504–10.
80. Achkar AA, Lie JT, Hunder GG, et al. How does previous corticosteroid treatment affect the biopsy findings in giant cell (temporal) arteritis? Ann Intern Med 1994;120:987–92.
81. Hoffman GS, Cid MC, Hellman D, et al. A multicenter, randomized, double-blind, placebo-controlled trial of adjuvant methotrexate treatment for giant cell arteritis. Arthritis Rheum 2002;46:1309–18.
82. Hoffman GS, Cid MC, Rendt-Zagar KE, et al. Infliximab for maintenance of glucocorticosteroid-induced remission of giant cell arteritis: a randomized trial. Ann Intern Med 2007;146:621–30.
83. Nesher G, Berkun Y, Mates M, et al. Low-dose aspirin and prevention of cranial ischemic complications in giant cell arteritis. Arthritis Rheum 2004;50:1332–7.
84. Lee MS, Smith SD, Galor A, et al. Antiplatelet and anticoagulant therapy in patients with giant cell arteritis. Arthritis Rheum 2006;54:3306–9.
85. Salvarani C, Cantini F, Boiardi L, et al. Polymyalgia rheumatica. Best Pract Res Clin Rheumatol 2004;18:705–22.
86. Gonzalez-Gay MA, Garcia-Porrua C, Salvarani C, et al. The spectrum of conditions mimicking polymyalgia rheumatica in Northwestern Spain. J Rheumatol 2000;27(9):2179–84.
87. Brooks RC, McGee SR. Diagnostic dilemmas in polymyalgia rheumatica. Arch Intern Med 1997;157:162–8.
88. Salvarani C, Cantini F, Olivieri I, et al. Proximal bursitis in active polymyalgia rheumatica. Ann Intern Med 1997;127:27–31.
89. Cantini F, Salvarani C, Olivieri I, et al. Shoulder ultrasonography in the diagnosis of polymyalgia rheumatica: a case-control study. J Rheumatol 2001;28: 1049–55.
90. Myklebust G, Gran JT. A prospective study of 287 patients with polymyalgia rheumatica and temporal arteritis: clinical and laboratory manifestations at onset of disease and at the time of diagnosis. Br J Rheumatol 1996;35(11): 1161–8.
91. Rynes RI, Mika P, Bartholomew LE. Development of giant cell (temporal) arteritis in a patient "adequately" treated for polymyalgia rheumatica. Ann Rheum Dis 1977;36:88–90.
92. Hernandez-Rodriguez J, Cid MC, Lopez-Soto A, et al. Treatment of polymyalgia rheumatica. Arch Intern Med 2009;169(20):1839–50.
93. Salvarani C, Cantini F, Niccoli L, et al. Treatment of refractory polymyalgia rheumatica with infliximab: a pilot study. J Rheumatol 2003;30:760–3.
94. Catanoso MG, Macchioni P, Boiardi L, et al. Treatment of refractory polymyalgia rheumatica with etanercept: an open pilot study. Arthritis Rheum 2007;57(8): 1514–9.

95. Corrao S, Pistone G, Scaglione R, et al. Fast recovery with etanercept in patients affected by polymyalgia rheumatica and decompensated diabetes: a case-series study. Clin Rheumatol 2009;28(1):89–92.
96. Salvarani C, Macchioni P, Manzini C, et al. Infliximab plus prednisone or placebo plus prednisone for the initial treatment of polymyalgia rheumatica. Ann Intern Med 2007;146(9):631–9.
97. Wolfe F, Smyth HA, Yunus MB, et al. The American College of Rheumatology 1990 criteria for the classification of fibromyalgia. Report of the Multicenter Criteria Committee. Arthritis Rheum 1990;33(2):160–72.
98. Weir PT, Harlan GA, Nkoy FL, et al. The incidence of fibromyalgia and its associated comorbidities: a population-based retrospective cohort study based on International Classification of Diseases, 9th Revision codes. J Clin Rheumatol 2006;12(3):124–8.
99. Watson NF, Buchwald D, Goldberg J, et al. Neurologic signs and symptoms in fibromyalgia. Arthritis Rheum 2009;60(9):2839–44.
100. Chervin RD, Teodorescu M, Kushwaha R, et al. Objective measures of disordered sleep in fibromyalgia. J Rheumatol 2009;36(9):2009–16.
101. Cole JA, Rothman KJ, Cabral HJ, et al. Migraine, fibromyalgia and depression among people with IBS: a prevalence study. BMC Gastroenterol 2006; 6:26.
102. Glass JM. Cognitive dysfunction in fibromyalgia and chronic fatigue syndrome: new trends and future directions. Curr Rheumatol Rep 2006;8(6):425–9.
103. Coury F, Rossat A, Tebib A, et al. Rheumatoid arthritis and fibromyalgia: a frequent unrelated association complicating disease management. J Rheumatol 2009;36(1):58–62.
104. Almansa C, Rey E, Sanchez RG, et al. Prevalence of functional gastrointestinal disorders in patients with fibromyalgia and the role of psychologic distress. Clin Gastroenterol Hepatol 2009;7(4):438–45.
105. Yunus MB. Fibromyalgia and overlapping disorders: the unifying concept of central sensitivity syndromes. Semin Arthritis Rheum 2007;36(6):339–56.
106. Aydin G, Basar MM, Keles I, et al. Relationship between sexual dysfunction and psychiatric status in premenopausal women with fibromyalgia. Urology 2006; 67(1):156–61.
107. Hassett AL, Gevirtz RN. Nonpharmacologic treatment for fibromyalgia: patient education, cognitive-behavioral therapy, relaxation techniques, and complementary and alternative medicine. Rheum Dis Clin North Am 2009;35(2): 393–407.
108. Hauser W, Bernardy K, Arnold B, et al. Efficacy of multicomponent treatment in fibromyalgia syndrome: a meta-analysis of randomized controlled clinical trials. Arthritis Rheum 2009;61(2):216–24.
109. Bennett RM, Kamin M, Karim R, et al. Tramadol and acetaminophen combination tablets in the treatment of fibromyalgia pain: a double-blind, randomized, placebo-controlled study. Am J Med 2003;114(7):537–45.
110. Hauser W, Bernardy K, Uceyler N, et al. Treatment of fibromyalgia syndrome with antidepressants: a meta-analysis. JAMA 2009;301(2):198–209.
111. Uceyler N, Hauser W, Sommer C. A systematic review on the effectiveness of treatment with antidepressants in fibromyalgia syndrome. Arthritis Rheum 2008;59(9):1279–98.
112. Arnold LM, Goldenberg DL, Stanford SB, et al. Gabapentin in the treatment of fibromyalgia: a randomized, double-blind, placebo-controlled, multicenter trial. Arthritis Rheum 2007;56(4):1336–44.

113. Crofford LJ, Mease PJ, Simpson SL, et al. Fibromyalgia relapse evaluation and efficacy for durability of meaningful relief (FREEDOM): a 6-month, double-blind, placebo-controlled trial with pregabalin. Pain 2008;136(3):419–31.
114. Russell IJ, Mease PJ, Smith TR, et al. Efficacy and safety of duloxetine for treatment of fibromyalgia in patients with or without major depressive disorder: results from a 6-month, randomized, double-blind, placebo-controlled, fixed-dose trial. Pain 2008;136(3):432–44.
115. Mease PJ, Clauw DJ, Gendreau RM, et al. The efficacy and safety of milnacipran for treatment of fibromyalgia. A randomized, double-blind, placebo-controlled trial. J Rheumatol 2009;36(2):398–409.
116. Tomas-Carus P, Gusi N, Hakkinen A, et al. Eight months of physical training in warm water improves physical and mental health in women with fibromyalgia: a randomized controlled trial. J Rehabil Med 2008;40(4):248–52.
117. Busch AJ, Schachter CL, Overend TJ, et al. Exercise for fibromyalgia: a systematic review. J Rheumatol 2008;35(6):1130–44.
118. Bircan C, Karasel SA, Akgun B, et al. Effects of muscle strengthening versus aerobic exercise program in fibromyalgia. Rheumatol Int 2008;28(6):527–32.
119. Sephton SE, Salmon P, Weissbecker I, et al. Mindfulness meditation alleviates depressive symptoms in women with fibromyalgia: results of a randomized clinical trial. Arthritis Rheum 2007;57(1):77–85.
120. Martin DP, Sletten CD, Williams BA, et al. Improvement in fibromyalgia symptoms with acupuncture: results of a randomized controlled trial. Mayo Clin Proc 2006;81(6):749–57.
121. Lucas N, Macaskill P, Irwig L, et al. Reliability of physical examination for diagnosis of myofascial trigger points: a systematic review of the literature. Clin J Pain 2009;25(1):80–9.
122. Hong CZ. Treatment of myofascial pain syndrome. Curr Pain Headache Rep 2006;10(5):345–9.
123. Fernandez-de-Las-Penas C, Alonso-Blanco C, Cuadrado ML, et al. Myofascial trigger points and their relationship to headache clinical parameters in chronic tension-type headache. Headache 2006;46(8):1264–72.
124. Majlesi J, Unalan H. Effect of treatment on trigger points. Curr Pain Headache Rep 2010;14(5):353–60.
125. Vernon H, Schneider M. Chiropractic management of myofascial trigger points and myofascial pain syndrome: a systematic review of the literature. J Manipulative Physiol Ther 2009;32(1):14–24.
126. Ay S, Evcik D, Tur BS. Comparison of injection methods in myofascial pain syndrome: a randomized controlled trial. Clin Rheumatol 2010;29(1):19–23.
127. Venâncio Rde A, Alencar FG, Zamperini C. Different substances and dry-needling injections in patients with myofascial pain and headaches. Cranio 2008;26(2):96–103.
128. Yoon SH, Rah UW, Sheen SS, et al. Comparison of 3 needle sizes for trigger point injection in myofascial pain syndrome of the upper-and middle-trapezius muscle: a randomized controlled trial. Arch Phys Med Rehabil 2009;90(8):1332–9.
129. Borg-Stein J. Treatment of fibromyalgia, myofascial pain, and related disorders. Phys Med Rehabil Clin N Am 2006;17(2):491–510.
130. Tüzün EH, Albayrak G, Eker L, et al. A comparison study of quality of life in women with fibromyalgia and myofascial pain syndrome. Disabil Rehabil 2004;26(4):198–202.

Conservative Treatment for Neck Pain: Medications, Physical Therapy, and Exercise

Sanjog Pangarkar, MD[a,c], Paul C. Lee, MD[b,c],*

KEYWORDS

- Neck pain • Medications • Exercise • Physical therapy
- Modalities

This article offers conservative treatment strategies for patients suffering from musculoskeletal causes of neck pain. Basic pharmacology is reviewed, including that of opioids, nonsteroidal anti-inflammatory drugs (NSAIDs), adjuvants, and topical analgesics. Moreover, indications for therapeutic exercise, manual therapy, and modalities are reviewed, along with any supporting literature. Treatment considerations with each category of medication and physical therapy are discussed. This article is meant to serve as a resource for physicians to tailor conservative treatment options to their individual patients.

MEDICATIONS

Recommendations of the World Health Organization (WHO) can help guide clinical decision making regarding appropriate medications for the patient with neck pain. These are organized into a conceptual stepladder (**Box 1**).

The first step of the ladder involves the use of nonopioid medications and adjuvant medications. Nonopioid medications typically include acetaminophen and NSAIDs,

Nothing to disclaim and no source of grant money.

[a] Inpatient Pain Service, Veterans Health Service Greater Los Angeles, David Geffen School of Medicine at UCLA, 11301 Wilshire Boulevard, Los Angeles, CA 90073, USA

[b] UCLA/VA Greater Los Angeles Multicampus Physical Medicine and Rehabilitation Residency Program, 11301 Wilshire Boulevard, Los Angeles, CA 90073, USA

[c] Department of Physical Medicine and Rehabilitation, VA Greater Los Angeles, Room 117, 11301 Wilshire Boulevard, Los Angeles, CA 90073, USA

* Corresponding author. Department of Physical Medicine and Rehabilitation, VA Greater Los Angeles, 11301 Wilshire Boulevard, Los Angeles, CA 90073.

E-mail address: Lee.Paul.C@gmail.com

Phys Med Rehabil Clin N Am 22 (2011) 503–520
doi:10.1016/j.pmr.2011.04.001
1047-9651/11/$ – see front matter

Box 1
WHO analgesic stepladder

Step 1

- Nonopioid medications: ± Adjuvants
  - Tylenol
  - NSAIDs

Step 2

- Add "weak" opioid for moderate pain: ± Adjuvants
  - Acetaminophen + Codeine
  - Acetaminophen + Oxycodone
  - Acetaminophen + Hydrocodone

Step 3

- Start "strong" opioid: ie, ± Adjuvants
  - Morphine
  - Dilaudid
  - Methadone
  - Oxycodone
  - Fentanyl

Data from World Health Organization. Cancer pain relief. 2nd edition. Geneva (Switzerland): World Health Organization, 2002.

---

whereas adjuvant medications include certain antidepressants, antiepileptics, and muscle relaxants. If the use of step 1 strategies does not satisfactorily manage the patient's pain, the next step of the WHO analgesic ladder is the addition or substitution of a "weak" opioid. This category includes hydrocodone or oxycodone + acetaminophen. Dosing of opiate + acetaminophen medications are limited by the maximum allowable amount of acetaminophen in a 24-hour period. Similarly, if these do not satisfactorily control a patient's pain, WHO recommendations for step 3 are the advent of "strong" opioids. Medications considered "strong" opioids are morphine, oxycodone, fentanyl, oxymorphone, and methadone.

Nonsteroidal Anti-Inflammatories

NSAIDs are on the first step of the WHO analgesic ladder (**Table 1**). NSAIDS reduce inflammation by blocking prostaglandin production through the inhibition of cyclooxygenase enzymes, COX-1 and COX-2, in the prostaglandin production pathway.[1,2] Most anti-inflammatory actions of NSAIDs are attributable to inhibition of COX-2, whereas many of the unwanted side effects are attributable to inhibition of COX-1. Traditional NSAIDs inhibit both COX-1 and COX-2, thereby reducing pain and inflammation but also predisposing to unwanted gastrointestinal (GI) side effects. The cumulative risk for serious adverse GI events increases over time. Risk factors for serious GI events are age, corticosteroid use, high NSAID dose, disability level, and previous NSAID-induced GI symptoms.[3] Medications more selective of COX-2 inhibition such as celecoxib and meloxicam have fewer GI side effects because gastric production of cytoprotective prostacyclin through the COX-1 pathway is preserved. Although

Table 1 Categories of nonsteroidal anti-inflammatory drugs		
Salicylates	Aspirin Salsalate Diflunisal	
Propionic Acids	Ibuprofen Naproxen Fenoprofen Ketoprofen Flurbiprofen Oxaprozin	
Acetic Acids	Arylalkanoic acids	Diclofenac Indomethacin Sulindac Tolmetin
	Pyrroles	Ketorolac
	Pyranocarboxylic acids	Etodalac
	Napthylalkanones	Nabumetone
Enolic Acids	Meloxicam Piroxicam	
Fenamic Acids	Meclofenamate Mefenamic acid	
Selective Cox-2 Inhibitors	Celecoxib	
Sulphonanilides	Nimesulide	
Pyrazolidinediones	Phenylbutazone	

these medications have been shown to have fewer GI side effects when compared with traditional NSAIDs,[4] some COX-2 inhibitors are associated with increased cardiovascular risk.[5] Recently, COX-2 inhibitors valdecoxib (Bextra) and rofecoxib (Vioxx) were removed from the US market; Bextra was shown to have increased potential for Stevens Johnson syndrome and increased mortality in patients with coronary artery bypass grafts[6–8] and Vioxx was shown to have increased overall cardiac mortality.[9] In addition, a 2006 meta-analysis by Singh and colleagues[10] suggested that some nonselective NSAIDs such as diclofenac and ibuprofen also increase the risk of adverse cardiovascular events, such as myocardial infarction. Other nonselective NSAIDs, such as naproxen, have been shown to have fewer adverse cardiovascular effects.[5]

Another significant adverse effect of NSAIDs is renal failure.[11] Caution is therefore advised in the elderly, as this population may have higher risk of GI bleed, cardiovascular disease, and impaired renal function.

Acetaminophen

Acetaminophen is another WHO step 1 analgesic medication commonly used to treat neck pain. The mechanism of action for acetaminophen is not clearly understood but is believed to be secondary to central antipyretic and analgesic actions activated by descending serotonergic pathways. Like NSAIDs, it is also known to inhibit prostaglandin synthesis; however, as only a weak inhibitor of COX-1 and COX-2, it has little anti-inflammatory activity. There has also been some discussion that inhibition of COX-3, a splice variant of COX-1, is involved,[12] but more recent analysis indicates that this interaction is not clinically relevant. Graham suggests that the primary site of action is inhibition of prostaglandin synthesis through production of reactive metabolites by the peroxidase function of COX-2.[13]

The primary concern for acetaminophen is hepatotoxicity. In fact, acetaminophen is the most common cause of acute liver failure in the United States and the United Kingdom, with a trend toward increasing incidence.[14] The maximum recommended dosage of acetaminophen for 24 hours is 4 g in divided doses. However, in 2009, the Food and Drug Administration Advisory Panel recommended decreasing the total daily dosage of acetaminophen to 3250 mg because of this risk (**Table 2**).[15,16] In fact, Watkins and colleagues[17] demonstrated that recurrent daily intake of 4 g of acetaminophen in healthy adults was associated with alanine aminotransferase elevations; patients with a history of depression, chronic pain, alcohol use, narcotic use, or who take several acetaminophen-based preparations simultaneously may be at higher risk for hepatotoxicity.[18] It is important to note that acetaminophen has also demonstrated renal toxicity with prolonged use.[19]

Opioids

There are 3 main types of opioid receptors: mu, delta, and kappa. The analgesic and side-effect profile of an opioid depends on how well it binds to a particular receptor.[20] For example, morphine preferentially binds mu-receptors over delta and kappa. Delta-receptor and kappa-receptor agonists have arguably lower abuse potential and side-effect burden than mu-opioid receptor agonists.[21]

Although initially intended for use in the cancer population, opioids are commonly prescribed for chronic noncancer pain, including neck pain, and may be effective for short-term pain relief. When deciding to use opioids to treat neck pain, one must weigh the potential for risk of abuse and dependence versus undertreatment of a patient's pain. The undertreatment of pain has led to the development of initiatives to increase awareness of and improve pain control. However, some argue that these efforts have led to an increase in opioid adverse drug reactions.[22]

Tolerance, the development of a diminished response to a drug after continued use, should also be considered. Opioid rotation is one strategy for managing tolerance and involves changing from one opioid to another to prevent an otherwise gradual increase

Table 2 Analgesic medications	
Drug	**Recommended Maximum Dose**
Acetaminophen	650 mg PO 5 × per day (3250 mg/24 h)
Ibuprofen	800 mg PO QID (3.2 g/24 hs)
Naproxen	500 mg PO BID (1 g/24 h)
Sulindac	200 mg PO BID (600 mg/24 h)
Indomethacin	50 mg PO TID (150 mg/24 h)
Salsalate	1500 mg BID (3 g/24 h)
Diclofenac	50 mg PO TID (150 mg/24 h)
Etodolac	500 mg PO BID (1000 mg/24 h)
Tolmentin	600 mg PO TID (1.8 g/24 h)
Tramadol	100 mg PO q6h (400 mg/24 h)
Celecoxib	100 BID (200 mg/24 h)
Meloxicam	15 mg PO daily (15 mg/24 h)

Abbreviations: BID, twice a day; PO, by mouth; q, every; QID, 4 times a day; TID, 3 times a day.

in opioid dosing over time. This strategy allows a lower comparative dose secondary to incomplete cross tolerance between opioids.[23] Another strategy to lower tolerance is periodic opiate holidays with restarting of medication at a lower dosage. Although opioid rotations and holidays depend on different factors contributing to an individual's response to a specific opioid, they remain important strategies to use in the management of chronic neck pain.

When treating neck pain with opiates, it is important to keep in mind the possibility of opioid-induced hyperalgesia (OIH). OIH occurs when treatment with opioids results in a lowering of pain threshold. The clinical picture may be similar to that of opioid tolerance, with worsening pain despite increasing opioid doses. Abnormal pain symptoms such as allodynia may occur concurrently. Clinicians should suspect OIH when opioid treatment becomes less efficacious, particularly in the context of unexplained new pain, diffuse allodynia, or changes in quality of pain compared with that previously observed.[24] The cause of OIH is unknown but is believed to be related to receptor desensitization via uncoupling of the receptor from G-proteins, upregulation of the cAMP pathway, and activation of the N-methyl-D-aspartate (NMDA)-receptor system, as well as descending facilitation.[25] OIH should be considered in patients undergoing neck surgery, as large doses of intraoperative mu-receptor agonists were found to increase postoperative pain and morphine consumption.[25] Treatment strategies for OIH are similar to those for tolerance, and include opioid dose reduction, opioid rotation, and transition to agents with NMDA receptor antagonism.[26]

Tramadol

Although not specifically mentioned, combination medications such as tramadol are considered by the authors to be between step 1 and step 2 of the WHO analgesic ladder. Although the exact mechanism through which patients find relief with tramadol is uncertain, it is known that tramadol has action on both mu-opioid receptor activation, and on serotonin and norepinephrine reuptake inhibition. Because of its mixed mechanism of action, tramadol can be considered for mild-moderate pain before using "weak" opioids. However, in rare instances tramadol has led to abuse and dependence,[27] and it carries warnings about renal failure, seizures, and potential serotonin syndrome when used with other serotonergic medications.[28,29]

ADJUVANT MEDICATIONS

Adjuvant medications are nonopioids originally intended for other purposes but provide significant pain relief. Among these are antiepileptics, antidepressants, and muscle relaxants.

Neuropathic pain, typically characterized by dysesthesias, burning pain, lancinating pain, and allodynia, can occur in the neck with conditions such as radiculopathy or myelopathy. Tricyclic antidepressants (TCAs), dual reuptake inhibitors of serotonin and norepinephrine, calcium channel alpha(2)-delta ligand agonists, and topical lidocaine were recommended as first-line treatment options as a result of randomized clinical trials.[30] In a 2007 study evaluating treatment options for peripheral neuropathic pain, the lowest identified number needed to treat was for tricyclic antidepressants, followed by opioids and the anticonvulsants gabapentin and pregabalin.[31]

After extensive study, TCAs have demonstrated efficacy against neuropathic pain. They may affect neuropathic pain by inhibiting presynaptic reuptake of serotonin and norepinephrine, but other mechanisms such as NMDA receptor and ion channel blockade are also thought to play a role. When using TCAs, it is necessary to consider their numerous contraindications, especially in patients with cardiovascular disease, owing to increased risks for conduction defects, arrhythmias, tachycardia, seizures, and stroke.[32] As such, one could consider obtaining a pretreatment electrocardiogram to rule out any concerning heart blocks or arrhythmias. Selective serotonin reuptake inhibitors have not proven to be as effective against neuropathic pain as TCAs.[33]

Antiepileptic drugs (AEDs) prevent seizures and improve neuropathic pain by raising the threshold for propagation of nerve impulses and depressing the potential for abnormal firing.[34,35] This is accomplished through interaction with various neurotransmitter receptors or ion channels, especially GABA-A receptors, sodium channels, and calcium channels. Multiple trials have demonstrated the safety and efficacy of alpha(2)-delta ligand agonists in treating neuropathic pain.[36] Gabapentin and pregabalin are commonly used AEDs. The mechanism of action of gabapentin is not completely defined, but it is thought that action on alpha(2)-delta voltage-dependent calcium channels influence GABAergic neurotransmission. Pregabalin is a structurally related medication with a similar mechanism of action that has been shown to reduce neuropathic pain from radiculopathy.[37,38] As these are adjunctive medications, it is not surprising that the combination of alpha(2)-delta ligand agonists and opioids is more effective in relief of neuropathic pain than either agent alone.[39]

Other AEDs, most of which were developed before 1980, appear to depress potential for abnormal neuronal discharges by acting on sodium channels, gamma-aminobutyric acid type A (GABA-A) receptors, or calcium channels. For example, benzodiazepines and barbiturates enhance GABA-A receptor-mediated inhibition; phenytoin, carbamazepine lamotrigine, oxcarbazepine, and possibly valproic acid work by enhancing sodium-channel inactivation; and ethosuximide and valproic acid reduce low-threshold calcium-channel current.[40] More research needs to be done to compare efficacy between AEDs in the treatment of neuropathic pain.

Muscle Relaxants

Skeletal muscle relaxants consist of antispasticity and antispasmodic agents. They are used to treat a variety of conditions from stroke-related spasticity and multiple sclerosis to musculoskeletal conditions such as muscle spasm and mechanical neck pain. Agents classified under antispasticity medications include baclofen, tizanidine, dantrolene, and diazepam. These are classically used for treating muscle hypertonicity and involuntary jerks. Antispasmodic agents, such as cyclobenzaprine, carisoprodol, methocarbamol, chlorzoxazone, and metaxalone, are primarily used to treat musculoskeletal conditions, such as muscle spasm and other myofascial pain. Although antispasmodic agents are often used for prolonged periods, their use in acute musculoskeletal injury ideally should not exceed 3 weeks, as evidence for prolonged use is not established. Although antispasmodic agents are seldom used to manage spasticity, either antispasticity agents or antispasmodic agents can be considered in the treatment of mechanical neck pain.

Efficacy of these medications with regard to spasticity will not be addressed given that musculoskeletal neck pain is the focus of this discussion. In this regard, cyclobenzaprine is the most studied and has been efficacious for various musculoskeletal conditions.[41] Cyclobenzaprine was found to be significantly better in treating neck and lumbar pain compared with diazepam.[42] Chou and colleagues[43] performed a systematic review of existing literature and concluded that there is fair evidence in favor of cyclobenzaprine, carisoprodol, orphenadrine, and tizanidine compared with placebo for patients with musculoskeletal neck pain, but limited or inconsistent data for metaxalone, methocarbamol, chlorzoxazone, baclofen, or dantrolene. However, there was insufficient evidence to determine safety or efficacy for these medications, and as such, treatment recommendations for these medications will depend on patient response, side effects, and cost. Tizanidine and cyclobenzaprine may benefit patients with insomnia caused by severe muscle spasms, whereas methocarbamol and metaxalone are less sedating but with weaker evidence of clinical effectiveness.[41] Common adverse effects of all muscle relaxants are dizziness and drowsiness. Dantrolene, and to a lesser degree chlorzoxazone, have been associated with rare but serious hepatotoxicity.[43]

One particular muscle relaxant that deserves special attention is carisoprodol. Although carisoprodol has a poorly understood mechanism of action, its effects are theorized to be related to the sedative properties of its metabolite, meprobamate. Unfortunately, meprobamate is known historically to have a high potential for dependence, abuse, and withdrawal. A literature review by Boothby and colleagues[44] produced little evidence to support the use of carisoprodol in pain control. It also showed that patients, especially those with a history of previous substance abuse, are more likely to abuse this drug. As there is little evidence to support efficacy and ample evidence to support abuse, clinicians should seriously consider the risk-benefit ratio before prescribing carisoprodol. In instances of withdrawal, other sedatives may be considered to alleviate symptoms.

TOPICAL ANALGESICS

Topical analgesics are pain-relieving agents applied directly onto the skin over painful areas of the body. There are 3 main types of topical analgesics: menthol/methylsalicylates, capsaicin, and anesthetics. Topical analgesics are absorbed through the skin and block local pain sensations.

Menthol elicits a cooling sensation over painful areas. Classically, menthol's analgesic properties were considered a result of gate control theory; the stimulation of sensory receptors to detect cold suppresses the perception of painful stimuli. More recently, it was discovered that low temperatures produce sensation of cold through action potentials generated by the activation of TRPM8 calcium channels, and that application of menthol has a similar effect on these channels.[45,46] TRPM8 receptors also stimulate small-diameter C and A-delta nerve fibers and affect the central nervous system through either endogenous opiates or glutamate receptors in the spinal cord.[47,48] One study suggests that these receptors may also have action on kappa-opioid receptors.[49]

Topical capsaicin has also been shown to decrease neck pain.[50] Capsaicin, structurally known as 8-methyl-N-vanillyl-6-nonenamide, produces topical analgesia by desensitizing pain fibers and eliciting a sensation of heat at the skin. It does this by selectively binding to TRPV1, a heat-activated calcium channel on the membranes of pain-sensing and heat-sensing neurons.[51] The TRPV1 receptor is activated between temperatures of 37 and 45°C. Capsaicin causes the channel to open below 37°C, resulting in an influx of calcium and producing a sensation of heat. With repeated exposure to capsaicin, C-fiber sensory neurons become depleted of substance P, a principal neurotransmitter of nociceptive impulses, resulting in analgesia. Topical capsaicin is not associated with notable systemic adverse effects, but severe burning of the skin at the site of application has been reported in almost 80% of patients. This effect often decreases with repeated use, but may interfere with compliance.[52] A review of capsaicin use in chronic musculoskeletal or neuropathic pain showed moderate to poor efficacy, and recommended its use in patients unresponsive or intolerant to other treatments.[53]

Topical versions of local anesthetics are also used to treat pain. Anesthetics such as lidocaine relieve pain by blocking the sodium channels necessary for nerves to transmit pain signals.[54] Studies have shown these to be effective in treating pain associated with neuropathy, venipuncture, surgery, and biopsies.[55–58]

The advantages of topical agents include targeted pain relief, less systemic absorption, and lower risk of adverse side effects. However, it is important to avoid contact with eyes and open wounds when using these agents.

Trigger Point Injections

Local injections allow placement of medication directly at the location where its action is most desired. Commonly used medications are local anesthetics, corticosteroids, and botulinum toxin. Injection of lidocaine into myofascial trigger points has been shown to improve visual analog pain scores and quality of life.[59] One study found that intramuscular injection of lidocaine for chronic mechanical neck pain was superior to placebo or dry needling in the short term.[60] However, another recent study comparing local anesthetic to dry needling of trigger points found statistically significant improvements in visual analog pain scale, cervical range of motion, and Beck Depression Inventory scores with both treatments.[61] In addition, a prospective randomized evaluation of treatments for myofascial trigger points argues that dry needling provides as much relief as when a local anesthetic or corticosteroid is injected.[62] Given this uncertainty and lack of consensus in the literature, one should weigh the risks and benefits when using trigger point injections for myofascial pain.

Botulinum toxin is another injectable agent used to treat mechanical and myofascial pain. It works by inhibiting presynaptic acetylcholine release. Although one study showed that injection of botulinum toxin improves visual analog pain scores and quality of life measures compared with dry needling in myofascial disorders,[59] it has not been shown to be superior to saline injection for chronic mechanical neck disorders.[60,63] Injection of botulinum toxin was also comparable to local anesthetic in terms of duration and degree of pain relief, function, and patient satisfaction.[64] In a review of 5 clinical trials, only one study concluded that botulinum toxin was effective, whereas the others did not support its utility in reducing trigger point pain.[65] Still, some consider injection of botulinum toxin as a second-line treatment when patients fail to achieve adequate relief with other modalities. Other important considerations with botulinum toxin are its cost and risk of dysphagia, particularly when injecting in the cervical regions.

PHYSICAL MODALITIES

The purpose of any treatment modality is to facilitate therapeutic activity and functional ability (**Box 2**). Therapeutic exercises, manual therapy, electrotherapy, thermal modalities, and even mechanical traction are commonly used for the conservative treatment of neck pain. Although there are numerous studies exploring therapy in the treatment of neck pain, clear undisputed evidence of benefit does not yet exist.[66]

Therapeutic Exercise

Therapeutic exercise is widely used as part of comprehensive conservative management of neck pain. Postural evaluation, support, and therapeutic exercises are considered by some to be a foundation of treatment. Patients may have aberrations in head and neck posture, such as abnormal cervical curvature and forward head carriage. Cervical curvature can be assessed visually, as well as on C-spine x-rays. Forward head carriage can be detected when the tragus of the ear lies anterior to the tip of the acromion. These postural habits are believed to contribute to development of cervical muscle imbalance and consequent mechanical neck pain.[67] Postural awareness and adjustment exercises based on strengthening, stretching, and range of motion may be helpful. In addition, ergonomic evaluation and modification of workstations may help prevent postural issues and subsequent neck pain.

Box 2
Modalities used in treatment of neck pain

Manual interventions:

- Orthoses
- Massage
- Mobilization
- Manipulation
- Traction

Electrical treatment:

- Galvanic stimulation
- Interferential current
- Microcurrent
- Transcutaneous electrical nerve stimulation (TENS)
- Neuromuscular stimulation

Thermal modalities:

- Therapeutic ultrasound
- Diathermy
- Heating pads (dry or moist)
- Infrared light
- Hydrotherapy
- Ice pack with or without massage
- Spray and spray and stretch

A study by Chiu and colleagues[68] concluded that patients with chronic neck pain benefit from exercise with significant improvement in disability, pain, and isometric neck muscle strength in the short term, but not necessarily at 6 months. However, in a review article, Gross and colleagues[69] cited moderate evidence to support long-term functional improvement after strengthening and stretching programs for chronic mechanical neck disorders. In a study involving women with chronic neck pain, Ylinen and colleagues[70] concluded that the inclusion of strength and endurance training with a stretching and aerobic exercising program over 12 months was effective in decreasing pain and disability. Neck stabilization exercises alone did not appear to provide benefit over a general physical therapy program for neck pain.[71] In a Cochrane review of 31 selected trials, Kay and colleagues[72] concluded that there is moderate evidence supporting focused stretching and strengthening at the cervical, shoulder, and thoracic regions for improving pain in chronic mechanical neck disorders. Their findings also suggest that strengthening exercises alone help to reduce mechanical neck pain and improve function, although they found no evidence of differences between the different exercise approaches.

Manual Therapy

Manual therapy is the physical application of force to the muscles and joints of the neck and body. It includes, but is not limited to, techniques such as massage, soft tissue mobilization, myofascial release, mobilization of joints, joint manipulation, mobilization of neural tissue, and the strain/counterstrain technique.

A number of studies have demonstrated varying amounts of efficacy of manual therapy. In one study, a manual therapy and exercise program resulted in significant short-term and long-term improvements in pain, disability, and patient-perceived recovery in patients with mechanical neck pain when compared with a program consisting of advice, exercise, and subtherapeutic ultrasound.[73] In another study, pain and disability scores slightly favored manual therapy over other methods of physical therapy and over continued care by a general practitioner.[74] In a follow-up study, manual therapy improved recovery time when compared with care from a general practitioner, and, to a lesser extent, with other methods of physical therapy at short-term follow-up (7 weeks). However, these differences were not sustained over longer follow-up periods (13-week and 52-week follow-up).[75] Miller and colleagues[76] supported this conclusion in a separate study with similar findings suggesting greater short-term pain relief with manual therapy than with exercise alone, but no long-term differences across multiple outcomes for neck pain. Kay and colleagues[72] noted that the strongest evidence for pain relief was with a multimodal approach that used exercise along with mobilization or manipulation. A review by Gross and colleagues[69] also supported this conclusion.

Traction

Cervical traction is often used in the management of neck pain as a means of spinal decompression. Gentle traction is theorized to relieve pressure on anatomic structures in the neck that may be a source of pain, such as pinched nerve roots and disc herniations. It is often performed as part of manual therapy by a therapist or chiropractor. There are also devices of varying costs and unproven efficacy, such as motorized equipment or gravity devices.

Current evidence regarding cervical traction is mixed. A study by Joghataei and colleagues[77] showed that the addition of mechanical intermittent cervical traction to a regimen of ultrasound and exercise improved patient grip strength compared with those who received only ultrasound and exercise therapy. In another small study, 24 of 26 patients with cervical disc herniations avoided surgery after treatment with both traction and cervical exercise.[78] However, a randomized study by Borman and colleagues[79] demonstrated no benefit of traction over standard physiotherapeutic interventions in adults with chronic neck pain. In addition, a randomized clinical trial by Young and colleagues[80] concluded that there was no significant additional benefit with regard to pain, function, or disability when adding mechanical cervical traction to other manual therapy and exercise in patients with cervical radiculopathy.

Despite these mixed results, traction continues to be used in the treatment of cervical pain. In light of this, the physician should be aware of absolute contraindications to traction, including osteoporosis, cervical infections or malignancies, cervical vascular insufficiency, and history of ligamentous instability or connective tissue disorders, such as rheumatoid arthritis.

Electrotherapy

Electrotherapy is the application of electrical energy to muscles and soft tissues to treat pain. Electrotherapy is theorized to work via the gate control theory of pain,[81] but has also been shown to promote release of endorphins.[82,83] In relation to neck pain, types of electrotherapy include transcutaneous electrical nerve stimulator (TENS) units, interferential current, galvanic stimulation, and iontophoresis.

A TENS unit is a small portable stimulator that allows for high-frequency (60–200 Hz) or low-frequency (<10 Hz) stimulation through adhesive pads placed over painful areas of the body. Higher-frequency settings produce shorter pain relief with longer application. Lower-frequency settings are more uncomfortable and not as well tolerated over long periods, but resultant pain relief can be longer in duration. The benefits of TENS may not be immediate, and may require continued use over time to produce effective pain relief. Some studies have shown that TENS units can produce improvements in disability, strength, and pain,[84] whereas others concluded that TENS may have effectiveness over placebo but not necessarily over other interventions.[85] Side effects are rare and often minor, but include burns with prolonged application, skin irritation from the adhesive pads, and transient pain.

Interferential current (IFC) is a method to deliver stimulation deeper into tissue. It uses a higher frequency than TENS units (4000 Hz). This higher frequency typically results in less discomfort for the user, and the waveforms travel deeper to deliver a TENS-like signal. In one study, use of interferential current alone did not demonstrate significant pain reduction over 3 months, but was effective when used as a supplement to other treatments compared with control treatment and placebo.[86] There are still only a limited number of studies and a few exploring use of IFC alone, and as such, any results should be considered with caution.

Galvanic stimulation uses direct current instead of the alternating current used in TENS and IFC units. Direct current is thought to create an electric field over tissues that theoretically reduces circulation to an area of acute injury, reduces swelling, and promotes healing. Unfortunately, studies regarding galvanic stimulation are also limited in quality and quantity. One Turkish study concluded galvanic stimulation combined with exercise was effective in the treatment of trigger-point tenderness when followed-up in the mid-term.[87] However, a more recent review concluded that galvanic stimulation is not able to reduce pain or disability and is not more effective than placebo.[85]

Iontophoresis is the use of electrical current to deliver medication through the skin into the tissue below. Corticosteroids, for example, are thought by some to travel deeper with iontophoresis. In a 2005 review of electrotherapy, Kroeling and colleagues[88] concluded that there was low-quality evidence that iontophoresis was more effective than placebo. However, in a follow-up study in 2009, they concluded that iontophoresis is not able to improve pain or disability.[85]

When treating neck pain with electrotherapy, the anterior regions of the neck or areas near the carotid vessels should be avoided. Application in this region may result in laryngospasm or a vasovagal reflex from stimulation of the carotid sinuses. TENS units may also interfere with pacemakers and implantable cardioverter defibrillator devices.[89–91] In addition, TENs should be avoided in pregnancy, over areas of known malignancy or infection, and over insensate skin. Overall, most studies on electrotherapy are low quality and have produced mixed results. Limitations in sample size and standardization will need to be addressed in future trials.

Thermal Modalities: Cryotherapy and Thermotherapy

Thermal modalities are safe, relatively inexpensive, easily applied, and have been shown to have some benefit in anecdotal, clinical, and physiologic research.[92] These modalities are thought to relieve neck pain by affecting nociception, local circulation, metabolism, and function of soft tissues.

Cryotherapy consists of the application of cold to relieve pain. This may include the use of ice packs, coolant sprays, or cold compression units. It is typically used in conjunction with other therapeutic techniques and exercise. Cryotherapy can be beneficial after exercise therapy, as it causes vasoconstriction and may decrease edema and inflammation.[93,94] However, one review argues that the addition of cryotherapy offers no additional benefit with regard to pain, swelling, and range of motion when compared with other rehabilitation methods used alone, and that more high-quality studies are required to guide the use of cryotherapy.[95,96]

Thermotherapy consists of the application of heat to relieve pain. Like cryotherapy, it is typically used in conjunction with other therapeutic techniques, such as exercise. Heat is theorized to cause vasodilation, thereby increasing tissue oxygenation and transport of metabolites to the tissue. Heat is also thought to alter viscoelastic properties of tissue leading to better soft tissue extensibility.

Thermotherapy can be further divided into superficial and deep heat modalities. Superficial heat modalities include warm compresses, paraffin baths, moist heat, infrared light, or whirlpool therapy. Although some studies suggest that superficial heat reduces pain and improves function in patients with musculoskeletal pain,[97] other analyses have argued that there is limited and insufficient evidence to support its use.[96,98]

Deep heat can be applied via the use of ultrasound and short wave diathermy. Ultrasound uses sound waves to deliver heat into the deeper tissues of the body. Several studies have demonstrated efficacy for ultrasound in the treatment of neck pain. One recent study showed benefit of ultrasound in softening trigger points and relieving pain in the trapezius area.[99] A randomized clinical trial concluded that therapeutic ultrasound has antinociceptive effects, reduces short-term trigger point sensitivity, and may be a useful treatment for trigger points and myofascial pain syndromes.[100,101] Similarly, a recent double-blind placebo-controlled study showed significant improvements in pain, disability, and quality-of-life parameters in patients with myofascial pain syndrome after ultrasound therapy.[102] These studies support ultrasound as a potential alternative or adjunct to injections and manual release in the treatment of trigger points and myofascial pain. However, ultrasound should be avoided in areas of infection, inflammation, or malignancy. In addition, patients suffering from cardiac disease should not receive treatment over the cervical ganglia, the stellate ganglion, the heart, or the vagus nerve, as a reflex coronary vasospasm might result. Treatment should also be avoided over anterior cervical structures, such as the carotid arteries, and in patients with history of cervical laminectomies or metallic implants.

Phonophoresis is the use of ultrasound to apply steroids or other medications in hopes of increasing their absorption deeper into tissues. It is analogous to iontophoresis. However, it remains questionable whether phonophoresis has benefits over ultrasound alone. One study showed that the rate of appearance and concentration of serum dexamethasone was greater in those receiving phonophoresis,[103] but a contrasting study showed that phonophoresis did not produce improved pain relief over ultrasound alone.[104] Despite conflicting studies, phonophoresis remains commonly used.

Shortwave diathermy is another thermal modality that delivers deep heat to tissues, and it does so via high-frequency electrical currents. As with many modalities, results are mixed. Some studies have reported that pulsed shortwave diathermy (PSWD) significantly reduced pain in patients with mechanical neck pain.[105,106] However, a randomized controlled trial by Dziedzic and colleagues[107] concluded that PSWD did not have significant improvements in neck pain when compared with advice and exercise alone. PSWD contraindications are similar to those of ultrasound: it should be avoided in areas of malignancy or sensory loss, over metal, and over inflammation. Currently, this modality is no longer used on a widespread basis.

As with superficial heat, questions remain whether there is sufficient evidence to support the use of deep heat modalities, such as ultrasound and shortwave diathermy.[98] Although the history of managing neck pain with thermal modalities is long, research has yet to yield unequivocal, supportive, evidence-based literature. However, these modalities are relatively low risk and inexpensive, and some patients find relief in their use.

SUMMARY

The conservative management of neck pain may consist of medications, exercise, physical therapy, and other modalities. Unfortunately, the subjective nature of neck pain and the lack of quality evidence for many modalities makes navigation of these treatment options difficult for both patient and physician. Ultimately, clinicians will have to individualize therapy based on etiology, symptoms, needs, and tolerances for a particular patient.

REFERENCES

1. Dubois RN, Abramson SB, Crofford L, et al. Cyclooxygenase in biology and disease. FASEB J 1998;12(12):1063–73.
2. Vane JR, Botting RM. Mechanism of action of nonsteroidal anti-inflammatory drugs. Am J Med 1998;104(3A):2S–8S [discussion: 21S–2S].
3. Singh G. Recent considerations in nonsteroidal anti-inflammatory drug gastropathy. Am J Med 1998;105(1B):31S–8S.
4. Strand V. Are COX-2 inhibitors preferable to non-selective non-steroidal anti-inflammatory drugs in patients with risk of cardiovascular events taking low-dose aspirin? Lancet 2007;370(9605):2138–51.
5. Fosbøl EL, Folke F, Jacobsen S, et al. Cause-specific cardiovascular risk associated with nonsteroidal antiinflammatory drugs among healthy individuals. Circ Cardiovasc Qual Outcomes 2010;3(4):395–405.
6. Ott E, Nussmeier NA, Duke PC, et al. Multicenter Study of Perioperative Ischemia (McSPI) Research Group, Ischemia Research and Education Foundation (IREF) Investigators. Efficacy and safety of the cyclooxygenase 2 inhibitors parecoxib and valdecoxib in patients undergoing coronary artery bypass surgery. J Thorac Cardiovasc Surg 2003;125(6):1481–92.
7. Nussmeier NA, Whelton AA, Brown MT, et al. Complications of the COX-2 inhibitors parecoxib and valdecoxib after cardiac surgery. N Engl J Med 2005; 352(11):1081–91.
8. La Grenade L, Lee L, Weaver J, et al. Comparison of reporting of Stevens-Johnson syndrome and toxic epidermal necrolysis in association with selective COX-2 inhibitors. Drug Saf 2005;28(10):917–24.
9. Jüni P, Nartey L, Reichenbach S, et al. Risk of cardiovascular events and rofecoxib: cumulative meta-analysis. Lancet 2004;364(9450):2021–9.
10. Singh G, Wu O, Langhorne P, et al. Risk of acute myocardial infarction with nonselective non-steroidal anti-inflammatory drugs: a meta-analysis. Arthritis Res Ther 2006;8(5):R153.
11. Perneger TV, Whelton PK, Klag MJ. Risk of kidney failure associated with the use of acetaminophen, aspirin, and nonsteroidal antiinflammatory drugs. N Engl J Med 1994;331(25):1675–9.
12. Botting RM. Mechanism of action of acetaminophen: is there a cyclooxygenase 3? Clin Infect Dis 2000;31(Suppl 5):S202–10.
13. Graham GG, Scott KF. Mechanism of action of paracetamol. Am J Ther 2005; 12(1):46–55.

14. Chun LJ, Tong MJ, Busuttil RW, et al. Acetaminophen hepatotoxicity and acute liver failure. J Clin Gastroenterol 2009;43(4):342–9.
15. Krenzelok EP. The FDA Acetaminophen Advisory Committee Meeting—what is the future of acetaminophen in the United States? The perspective of a committee member. Clin Toxicol (Phila) 2009;47(8):784–9.
16. Graham GG, Day RO, Graudins A, et al. FDA proposals to limit the hepatotoxicity of paracetamol (acetaminophen): are they reasonable? Inflammopharmacology 2010;18(2):47–55.
17. Watkins PB, Kaplowitz N, Slattery JT, et al. Aminotransferase elevations in healthy adults receiving 4 grams of acetaminophen daily: a randomized controlled trial. JAMA 2006;296(1):87–93.
18. Larson AM, Polson J, Fontana RJ, et al. Acute Liver Failure Study Group. Acetaminophen-induced acute liver failure: results of a United States multicenter, prospective study. Hepatology 2005;42(6):1364–72.
19. Curhan GC, Knight EL, Rosner B, et al. Lifetime nonnarcotic analgesic use and decline in renal function in women. Arch Intern Med 2004;164(14): 1519–24.
20. Przewlocki R, Przewlocka B. Opioids in chronic pain. Eur J Pharmacol 2001; 429(1–3):79–91.
21. Vanderah TW. Delta and kappa opioid receptors as suitable drug targets for pain. Clin J Pain 2010;26(Suppl 10):S10–5.
22. Vila H Jr, Smith RA, Augustyniak MJ, et al. The efficacy and safety of pain management before and after implementation of hospital-wide pain management standards: is patient safety compromised by treatment based solely on numerical pain ratings? Anesth Analg 2005;101(2):474–80.
23. Mercadante S. Opioid rotation for cancer pain: rationale and clinical aspects. Cancer 1999;86(9):1856–66.
24. Chu LF, Angst MS, Clark D. Opioid-induced hyperalgesia in humans: molecular mechanisms and clinical considerations. Clin J Pain 2008;24(6):479–96.
25. Koppert W. Opioid-induced hyperalgesia: pathophysiology and clinical relevance. Acute Pain 2007;9(1):21–4.
26. Mitra S. Opioid-induced hyperalgesia: pathophysiology and clinical implications. J Opioid Manag 2008;4(3):123–30.
27. Cicero TJ, Adams EH, Geller A, et al. A postmarketing surveillance program to monitor Ultram (tramadol hydrochloride) abuse in the United States. Drug Alcohol Depend 1999;57(1):7–22.
28. Desmeules JA. The tramadol option. Eur J Pain 2000;4(Suppl A):15–21.
29. Sansone RA, Sansone LA. Tramadol: seizures, serotonin syndrome, and coadministered antidepressants. Psychiatry (Edgmont) 2009;6(4):17–21.
30. Dworkin RH, O'Connor AB, Audette J, et al. Recommendations for the pharmacological management of neuropathic pain: an overview and literature update. Mayo Clin Proc 2010;85(Suppl 3):S3–14.
31. Finnerup NB, Otto M, Jensen TS, et al. An evidence-based algorithm for the treatment of neuropathic pain. MedGenMed 2007;9(2):36.
32. Dworkin RH, Backonja M, Rowbotham MC, et al. Advances in neuropathic pain: diagnosis, mechanisms, and treatment recommendations. Arch Neurol 2003; 60(11):1524–34.
33. Sindrup SH, Otto M, Finnerup NB, et al. Antidepressants in the treatment of neuropathic pain. Basic Clin Pharmacol Toxicol 2005;96(6):399–409.
34. Rogawski MA, Löscher W. The neurobiology of antiepileptic drugs for the treatment of nonepileptic conditions. Nat Med 2004;10(7):685–92.

35. Johannessen Landmark C. Antiepileptic drugs in non-epilepsy disorders: relations between mechanisms of action and clinical efficacy. CNS Drugs 2008;22(1):27–47.

36. Gilron I. Gabapentin and pregabalin for chronic neuropathic and early postsurgical pain: current evidence and future directions. Curr Opin Anaesthesiol 2007; 20(5):456–72.

37. Sills GJ. The mechanisms of action of gabapentin and pregabalin. Curr Opin Pharmacol 2006;6(1):108–13.

38. Saldaña MT, Navarro A, Pérez C, et al. Patient-reported-outcomes in subjects with painful lumbar or cervical radiculopathy treated with pregabalin: evidence from medical practice in primary care settings. Rheumatol Int 2010;30(8): 1005–15.

39. Gilron I, Bailey JM, Tu D, et al. Morphine, gabapentin, or their combination for neuropathic pain. N Engl J Med 2005;352(13):1324–34.

40. Macdonald RL, Kelly KM. Antiepileptic drug mechanisms of action. Epilepsia 1995;36(Suppl 2):S2–12.

41. See S, Ginzburg R. Choosing a skeletal muscle relaxant. Am Fam Physician 2008;78(3):365–70.

42. Basmajian JV. Cyclobenzaprine hydrochloride effect on skeletal muscle spasm in the lumbar region and neck: two double-blind controlled clinical and laboratory studies. Arch Phys Med Rehabil 1978;59(2):58–63.

43. Chou R, Peterson K, Helfand M. Comparative efficacy and safety of skeletal muscle relaxants for spasticity and musculoskeletal conditions: a systematic review. J Pain Symptom Manage 2004;28(2):140–75.

44. Boothby LA, Doering PL, Hatton RC. Carisoprodol: a marginally effective skeletal muscle relaxant with serious abuse potential. Hosp Pharm 2003;38:337–45.

45. Patapoutian A, Peier AM, Story GM, et al. ThermoTRP channels and beyond: mechanisms of temperature sensation. Nat Rev Neurosci 2003;4(7):529–39.

46. Baron R. Mechanisms of disease: neuropathic pain—a clinical perspective. Nat Clin Pract Neurol 2006;2(2):95–106.

47. Baron R. Neuropathic pain: a clinical perspective. Handb Exp Pharmacol 2009; 194:3–30.

48. Wasner G, Schattschneider J, Binder A, et al. Topical menthol—a human model for cold pain by activation and sensitization of C nociceptors. Brain 2004;127(Pt 5): 1159–71.

49. Galeotti N, Di Cesare Mannelli L, Mazzanti G, et al. Menthol: a natural analgesic compound. Neurosci Lett 2002;322(3):145–8.

50. Mathias BJ, Dillingham TR, Zeigler DN, et al. Topical capsaicin for chronic neck pain. A pilot study. Am J Phys Med Rehabil 1995;74(1):39–44.

51. Caterina MJ, Schumacher MA, Tominaga M, et al. The capsaicin receptor: a heat-activated ion channel in the pain pathway. Nature 1997;389(6653):816–24.

52. Argoff CE. Targeted topical peripheral analgesics in the management of pain. Curr Pain Headache Rep 2003;7(1):34–8.

53. Mason L, Moore RA, Derry S, et al. Systematic review of topical capsaicin for the treatment of chronic pain. BMJ 2004;328(7446):991.

54. Wood JN, Boorman JP, Okuse K, et al. Voltage-gated sodium channels and pain pathways. J Neurobiol 2004;61(1):55–71.

55. Rowbotham MC, Fields HL. Topical lidocaine reduces pain in post-herpetic neuralgia. Pain 1989;38(3):297–301.

56. Shavit I, Hadash A, Knaani-Levinz H, et al. Lidocaine-based topical anesthetic with disinfectant (LidoDin) versus EMLA for venipuncture: a randomized controlled trial. Clin J Pain 2009;25(8):711–4.

57. Gursoy A, Ertugrul DT, Sahin M, et al. The analgesic efficacy of lidocaine/prilocaine (EMLA) cream during fine-needle aspiration biopsy of thyroid nodules. Clin Endocrinol (Oxf) 2007;66(5):691–4.

58. Shiau JM, Su HP, Chen HS, et al. Use of a topical anesthetic cream (EMLA) to reduce pain after hemorrhoidectomy. Reg Anesth Pain Med 2008;33(1):30–5.

59. Kamanli A, Kaya A, Ardicoglu O, et al. Comparison of lidocaine injection, botulinum toxin injection, and dry needling to trigger points in myofascial pain syndrome. Rheumatol Int 2005;25(8):604–11.

60. Peloso P, Gross A, Haines T, et al. Cervical Overview Group. Medicinal and injection therapies for mechanical neck disorders. Cochrane Database Syst Rev 2007;3:CD000319.

61. Ay S, Evcik D, Tur BS. Comparison of injection methods in myofascial pain syndrome: a randomized controlled trial. Clin Rheumatol 2010;29(1):19–23.

62. Garvey TA, Marks MR, Wiesel SW. A prospective, randomized, double-blind evaluation of trigger-point injection therapy for low-back pain. Spine (Phila Pa 1976) 1989;14(9):962–4.

63. Ojala T, Arokoski JP, Partanen J. The effect of small doses of botulinum toxin a on neck-shoulder myofascial pain syndrome: a double-blind, randomized, and controlled crossover trial. Clin J Pain 2006;22(1):90–6.

64. Graboski CL, Gray DS, Burnham RS. Botulinum toxin A versus bupivacaine trigger point injections for the treatment of myofascial pain syndrome: a randomised double blind crossover study. Pain 2005;118(1/2):170–5.

65. Ho KY, Tan KH. Botulinum toxin A for myofascial trigger point injection: a qualitative systematic review. Eur J Pain 2007;11(5):519–27.

66. Borenstein DG. Chronic neck pain: how to approach treatment. Curr Pain Headache Rep 2007;11(6):436–9.

67. Edwards J. The importance of postural habits in perpetuating myofascial trigger point pain. Acupunct Med 2005;23(2):77–82.

68. Chiu TT, Lam TH, Hedley AJ. A randomized controlled trial on the efficacy of exercise for patients with chronic neck pain. Spine (Phila Pa 1976) 2005;30(1):E1–7.

69. Gross AR, Goldsmith C, Hoving JL, et al, Cervical Overview Group. Conservative management of mechanical neck disorders: a systematic review. J Rheumatol 2007;34(5):1083–102.

70. Ylinen J, Takala EP, Nykänen M, et al. Active neck muscle training in the treatment of chronic neck pain in women: a randomized controlled trial. JAMA 2003;289(19):2509–16.

71. Griffiths C, Dziedzic K, Waterfield J, et al. Effectiveness of specific neck stabilization exercises or a general neck exercise program for chronic neck disorders: a randomized controlled trial. J Rheumatol 2009;36(2):390–7.

72. Kay TM, Gross A, Goldsmith C, et al. Cervical Overview Group. Exercises for mechanical neck disorders. Cochrane Database Syst Rev 2005;3:CD004250.

73. Walker MJ, Boyles RE, Young BA, et al. The effectiveness of manual physical therapy and exercise for mechanical neck pain: a randomized clinical trial. Spine (Phila Pa 1976) 2008;33(22):2371–8.

74. Hoving JL, Koes BW, de Vet HC, et al. Manual therapy, physical therapy, or continued care by a general practitioner for patients with neck pain. A randomized, controlled trial. Ann Intern Med 2002;136(10):713–22.

75. Hoving JL, de Vet HC, Koes BW, et al. Manual therapy, physical therapy, or continued care by the general practitioner for patients with neck pain: long-term results from a pragmatic randomized clinical trial. Clin J Pain 2006;22(4):370–7.

76. Miller J, Gross A, D'Sylva J, et al. Manual therapy and exercise for neck pain: a systematic review. Man Ther 2010;15(4):334–54.

77. Joghataei MT, Arab AM, Khaksar H. The effect of cervical traction combined with conventional therapy on grip strength on patients with cervical radiculopathy. Clin Rehabil 2004;18:879–87. Available at: http://www.orthopt.org/ICF/ Neck Pain - Clinical Guideline - most recent.pdf. Accessed April 8, 2011.

78. Saal JS, Saal JA, Yurth EF. Nonoperative management of herniated cervical intervertebral disc with radiculopathy. Spine (Phila Pa 1976) 1996;21(16): 1877–83.

79. Borman P, Keskin D, Ekici B, et al. The efficacy of intermittent cervical traction in patents with chronic neck pain. Clin Rheumatol 2008;27(10):1249–53.

80. Young IA, Michener LA, Cleland JA, et al. Manual therapy, exercise, and traction for patients with cervical radiculopathy: a randomized clinical trial. Phys Ther 2009;89(7):632–42. Available at: http://www.physther.net/content/89/7/632.full. Accessed April 8, 2011.

81. Kroeling P, Gross AR, Goldsmith CH. Cervical Overview Group. A Cochrane review of electrotherapy for mechanical neck disorders. Spine (Phila Pa 1976) 2005;30(21):E641–8.

82. Salar G, Job I, Mingrino S, et al. Effect of transcutaneous electrotherapy on CSF beta-endorphin content in patients without pain problems. Pain 1981;10(2): 169–72.

83. Bender T, Nagy G, Barna I, et al. The effect of physical therapy on beta-endorphin levels. Eur J Appl Physiol 2007;100(4):371–82.

84. Chiu TT, Hui-Chan CW, Chein G. A randomized clinical trial of TENS and exercise for patients with chronic neck pain. Clin Rehabil 2005;19(8):850–60.

85. Kroeling P, Gross A, Goldsmith CH, et al. Electrotherapy for neck pain. Cochrane Database Syst Rev 2009;4:CD004251.

86. Fuentes JP, Armijo Olivo S, Magee DJ, et al. Effectiveness of interferential current therapy in the management of musculoskeletal pain: a systematic review and meta-analysis. Phys Ther 2010;90(9):1219–38.

87. Tanrikut A, Özaras N, Kaptan HA, et al. High voltage galvanic stimulation in myofascial pain syndrome. J Muscoskel Pain 2003;11(2):11–5.

88. Kroeling P, Gross A, Houghton PE, et al. Electrotherapy for neck disorders. Cochrane Database Syst Rev 2005;2:CD004251.

89. Philbin DM, Marieb MA, Aithal KH, et al. Inappropriate shocks delivered by an ICD as a result of sensed potentials from a transcutaneous electronic nerve stimulation unit. Pacing Clin Electrophysiol 1998;21(10):2010–1.

90. Pyatt JR, Trenbath D, Chester M, et al. The simultaneous use of a biventricular implantable cardioverter defibrillator (ICD) and transcutaneous electrical nerve stimulation (TENS) unit: implications for device interaction. Europace 2003;5(1): 91–3.

91. Holmgren C, Carlsson T, Mannheimer C, et al. Risk of interference from transcutaneous electrical nerve stimulation on the sensing function of implantable defibrillators. Pacing Clin Electrophysiol 2008;31(2):151–8.

92. Nanneman D. Thermal modalities: heat and cold. A review of physiologic effects with clinical applications. AAOHN J 1991;39(2):70–5.

93. MacAuley DC. Ice therapy: how good is the evidence? Int J Sports Med 2001; 22(5):379–84.

94. Swenson C, Swärd L, Karlsson J. Cryotherapy in sports medicine. Scand J Med Sci Sports 1996;6(4):193–200.

95. Hubbard TJ, Denegar CR. Does cryotherapy improve outcomes with soft tissue injury? J Athl Train 2004;39(3):278–9.
96. French SD, Cameron M, Walker BF, et al. A Cochrane review of superficial heat or cold for low back pain. Spine (Phila Pa 1976) 2006;31(9):998–1006.
97. Cetin N, Aytar A, Atalay A, et al. Comparing hot pack, short-wave diathermy, ultrasound, and TENS on isokinetic strength, pain, and functional status of women with osteoarthritic knees: a single-blind, randomized, controlled trial. Am J Phys Med Rehabil 2008;87(6):443–51.
98. Cohen SP, Argoff CE, Carragee EJ. Management of low back pain. BMJ 2008; 337:a2718.
99. Draper DO, Mahaffey C, Kaiser D, et al. Thermal ultrasound decreases tissue stiffness of trigger points in upper trapezius muscles. Physiother Theory Pract 2010;26(3):167–72.
100. Srbely JZ, Dickey JP, Lowerison M, et al. Stimulation of myofascial trigger points with ultrasound induces segmental antinociceptive effects: a randomized controlled study. Pain 2008;139(2):260–6.
101. Srbely JZ, Dickey JP. Randomized controlled study of the antinociceptive effect of ultrasound on trigger point sensitivity: novel applications in myofascial therapy? Clin Rehabil 2007;21(5):411–7.
102. Dündar Ü, Solak Ö, Şamlı S, et al. Effectiveness of ultrasound therapy in cervical myofascial pain syndrome: a double blind, placebo-controlled study. Turk J Rheumatol 2010;25:110–5.
103. Saliba S, Mistry DJ, Perrin DH, et al. Phonophoresis and the absorption of dexamethasone in the presence of an occlusive dressing. J Athl Train 2007;42(3): 349–54.
104. Klaiman MD, Shrader JA, Danoff JV, et al. Phonophoresis versus ultrasound in the treatment of common musculoskeletal conditions. Med Sci Sports Exerc 1998;30(9):1349–55.
105. Foley-Nolan D, Barry C, Coughlan RJ, et al. Pulsed high frequency (27MHz) electromagnetic therapy for persistent neck pain: a double blind, placebo-controlled study of 20 patients. Orthopedics 1990;13:445–51.
106. Foley-Nolan D, Moore K, Codd M, et al. Low energy high frequency pulsed electromagnetic therapy for acute whiplash injuries: a double blind randomized controlled study. Scand J Rehabil Med 1992;24:51–9.
107. Dziedzic K, Hill J, Lewis M, et al. Effectiveness of manual therapy or pulsed shortwave diathermy in addition to advice and exercise for neck disorders: a pragmatic randomized controlled trial in physical therapy clinics. Arthritis Care Res 2005;53:214–22.

Complementary and Alternative Treatment for Neck Pain: Chiropractic, Acupuncture, TENS, Massage, Yoga, Tai Chi, and Feldenkrais

Christopher T. Plastaras, MD[a],*, Seth Schran, MD[a],
Natasha Kim, DC[b], Susan Sorosky, MD[c], Deborah Darr, PT[d,e],
Mary Susan Chen, PT, GCFP[f], Rebecca Lansky, DO[a]

KEYWORDS

- CAM therapy • Acupuncture • Chiropractic • TENS • Yoga
- Tai Chi • Massage therapy • Feldenkrais

Neck pain is a modern American epidemic, affecting most adults at some time during their lives. In a survey of more than 2000 individuals, 54.2% of respondents experienced neck pain in the previous 6 months and neck pain disabled 4.6% of the adult population surveyed.[1] A 2007 National Health Interview Survey conducted by the Centers for Disease Control and Prevention's National Center for Health Statistics reported approximately 38% of adults and almost 12% of children used some form of complementary and alternative medicine therapy.[2] Although western medicine offers many options for the management of neck pain, most have modest efficacy at best and there are few with clearly demonstrated benefits. Therefore, many patients with chronic neck pain turn to complementary and alternative medicine (CAM)

[a] Department of Physical Medicine and Rehabilitation, Penn Spine Center, University of Pennsylvania, White Building, Ground Floor, 3400 Spruce Street, Philadelphia, PA 19104, USA
[b] Carmel, IN, USA
[c] Desert Spine and Sports Physicians, Phoenix, AZ 85018, USA
[d] Deborah Darr Physical Therapy, 900 North Lake Shore Drive, Suite 803, Chicago, IL 60611, USA
[e] Rehabilitation Institute of Chicago Center for Pain Management, 980 North Michigan Avenue, Suite 800, Chicago, IL 60611, USA
[f] Feldenkrais Guild of North America, Midwest Regional Representative, River Forest, IL, USA
* Corresponding author.
E-mail address: Christopher.plastaras@uphs.upenn.edu

Phys Med Rehabil Clin N Am 22 (2011) 521–537
doi:10.1016/j.pmr.2011.02.011
1047-9651/11/$ – see front matter © 2011 Elsevier Inc. All rights reserved.

pmr.theclinics.com

including chiropractic, acupuncture, transcutaneous electric nerve stimulation (TENS), massage, yoga, Tai Chi, and Feldenkrais to help manage their pain.

CHIROPRACTIC CARE

Since the beginnings of the chiropractic profession in the United States in 1895, there has been continued growth and interest in this therapeutic option. By the late 1990s, of the 42% of individuals using at least one form of alternative therapy within the past 12 months, 11.1% received chiropractic care.[3] Furthermore, nearly 8% of adults and 2.8% of children received chiropractic or osteopathic manipulative therapy in the prior 12 months.[2]

An important principle of chiropractic care involves functional reactivation of the patient. Whereas spinal manipulative therapy (SMT) remains a central feature of chiropractic care, this modality may be used in combination with rehabilitative exercises, ice, heat, electric stimulation, ultrasound, and encouragement of healthy lifestyle modifications. During the course of treatment, the gradual return to activity is encouraged. Ongoing reassessment helps ensure a path toward optimal recovery.[4]

The goals of SMT are to restore dysfunctional joint mechanics and to reduce mechanical stress on the adjacent tissues, thereby reducing pain. Three types of SMT have been described, including unloaded spinal motion, manual repetitive oscillations, and high velocity low amplitude (HVLA) manipulation. Unloaded spinal motion involves continuous passive motion with motorized tables and manual application of flexion-distraction techniques. HVLA manipulation is performed by delivering a quick, impulse-like thrust within a joint's range of motion. The chiropractor may choose a specific SMT technique considering such factors as the patient's age, stature, and diagnosis.[5]

Various theories have attempted to explain the benefits of chiropractic manipulation. Examples include the release of plica or entrapped synovial folds, the relaxation of hypertonic muscle by sudden stretch, the disruption of articular or periarticular adhesions, and the restoration of normal motion to displaced joints or vertebral segments.[6] The biomechanics of chiropractic manipulation have been well described by Triano.[5] Indications for SMT include focal tenderness to palpation, abnormal tissue tone, symptoms reproduced with provocative testing, and joint dysfunction or reduced mobility. Contraindications for SMT are listed in **Box 1**, including instability, infection, myelopathy, and so forth.[4]

Research has shown short-term treatment effect of SMT with exercise. A 2004 Cochrane review of mechanical neck disorders reported that mobilization and/or manipulation combined with exercise compared with no treatment led to improved function, pain reduction, and perceived effect.[7] A subsequent review of subacute and chronic neck pain reported that the combination of mobilization, manipulation, and exercise demonstrated greater short-term pain relief and quality of life improvements than exercise alone. Greater short-term pain reduction was also achieved in patients with acute whiplash with the combination of chiropractic treatment and exercise compared with traditional care, defined as any two of the following: cervical collar, advice, or pain medication. Radicular symptoms were not assessed.[8] Results from The Bone and Joint Decade (2000–2010) Task Force on Neck Pain and Associated Disorders showed education, mobilization, and exercise to be more efficacious than usual care or physical modalities for whiplash-associated disorders.[9]

Recent reviews have also demonstrated some benefits of SMT for neck disorders when used alone. A 2010 Cochrane review demonstrated "low-quality" evidence that neck manipulations for acute or chronic cervical conditions reduce pain in

Box 1
Contraindications to SMT

Relative contraindications

    Acute disk herniation

    Osteopenia

    Spondyloarthropathy

    Patient on anticoagulant medication

    Bleeding disorder

    Psychologic overlay

    Hypermobility

Absolute contraindications

    Progressive neurologic deficit

    Destructive lesions, malignancies

    Acute myelopathy

    Unstable os odontoideum

    Healing fracture or dislocation

    Avascular necrosis

    Bone infection

    Segmental instability

    Cauda equina syndrome

    Large abdominal aortic aneurysm

    Referred visceral pain

    Long-term repeated manipulation with symptom relief lasting less than 1 day

    Recognized secondary gain, malingering

Data from Liebenson C. Rehabilitation of the Spine. A practitioner's manual. Philadelphia: Lippincott Williams & Wilkins; 2007. p. 3–29; 72–90; 487–509; 753–75; 852–85.

comparison to controls. In addition, "very low to low-quality" evidence exists that thoracic spine manipulation alone provides immediate reduction in acute neck pain or whiplash symptoms.[10,11] Neck pain can be related to aberrant thoracic spine biomechanics, such as decreased thoracic spine mobility.[12] Thrust mobilization or manipulation showed greater short-term reduction in neck pain and disability than non-thrust technique.[13]

The most common side-effects of manipulation are generally benign and self-limited. In a prospective survey of 1058 patients undergoing 4712 treatments, the most common side-effects included local discomfort (53%), headache (12%), tiredness (11%), and radiating discomfort (10%). These effects tended to occur within 4 hours of treatment and were characterized as "mild" or "moderate" in the majority of patients. The majority experienced resolution within 24 hours without serious complications.[14] In a systematic review of SMT for neck pain, side-effects were also benign and transient, including radicular symptoms, headache, or exacerbation of neck pain.[10] The risk of minor symptoms appeared to be greater with manipulation versus mobilization in the report from the Bone and Joint Decade Task Force.[9] The risk of vertebrobasilar artery

(VBA) stroke has been estimated as 1 in 200,000[15] to 1 in several million.[16] A case-control study demonstrated that the risk of VBA stroke associated with chiropractic care was not significantly different than for primary care practitioners.[17]

Functional reactivation of the patient focuses on the patient's symptoms; dysfunction such as impairment, abilities, and participation in vocation and recreational activities; and distress. The goals of functional reactivation are to avoid inactivity, which can result in a deconditioned state, and to encourage a gradual, safe return to activities. Manual therapy, including SMT, is an integral part of chiropractic care that may be used alone or in combination with rehabilitative exercise, ice or heat, electric stimulation and ultrasound, and modification of lifestyle factors. The decision to apply SMT for the management of neck pain is a multifactorial process based on history, physical examination, and clinical assessment of the benefit to risk relationship in the context of patient preference.

ACUPUNCTURE

Acupuncture involves the insertion of needles into the body to achieve a treatment effect. Needle types and sizes vary, as do the techniques and theories behind their application. In the classical context, needles are inserted into well-defined, anatomic points on the body with the goal of influencing and normalizing the circulation of chi energy. The Chinese character for chi (also spelled qi) is translated as "rice vapor," and represents an energy gleaned from digested food and inspired air. Each person is bestowed with a certain amount of original energy at birth as well. Depending on the subtype of chi, it can flow around the body's surface to defend against external pathogens, along deeper channels or meridians, or from organ to organ in a cyclical pattern. Any imbalances in this flow, whether due to deficiency, excess, or blockage of chi, can result in disease states.

Using acupuncture needles, deficient chi can be tonified, excess chi can be dispersed, and obstructed chi can be dispelled with a series of treatments. Tonification of chi begins by inserting needles along the acupuncture points involving the deficient meridian or organ. Needle insertion is followed by one or more methods of tonification, including manipulating the needles manually, holding a burning, glowing moxa herb (*Artemmisia vulgaris*) near the inserted needles, or by applying low frequency (eg, 4 Hz) electrical stimulation via electrodes clipped to the needles. Dispersion of excess chi can be accomplished by leaving the inserted needles in place undisturbed. Obstructions in the flow of chi can be dispelled by inserting needles along the channel before and after the obstruction. High-frequency electrical stimulation can be applied to augment the effect. Some practitioners may also use herbal medicines, either alone or concurrent with acupuncture treatments, to further influence and harmonize chi.

Acupuncture can employ other paradigms besides influencing chi flow through channels and meridians. Ah Shi points, which are defined by the site of maximal tenderness to palpation rather than by anatomic landmarks, can be needled with the goal of reducing pain. The Japanese surface release technique involves insertion of numerous superficial needles over the affected area, with the idea that the effect penetrates to deeper levels. In auricular acupuncture and Korean hand acupuncture, the body as a whole is represented somatotopically on the ears or the hands, respectively. Local needles inserted into these somatotopic microsystems are thought to have therapeutic effects on the part of the body that is represented at the needle tip. These microsystems can be used alone or at the same time as other treatments to enhance the overall effect.

The heterogeneity of acupuncture interventions and difficulty in blinding present a challenge for reviewing the use of acupuncture for mechanical neck disorders (MND). Birch and Jamison[18] (1998) compared Japanese-style shallow needling of relevant points with sham treatment needling irrelevant points in patients with mechanical neck disorders. A significant treatment benefit was measured. White and colleagues[19] (2000) compared an acupuncture treatment involving needle insertion and stimulation to a sham treatment without needle stimulation and again found a treatment benefit measured at the end of the treatment. However, while showing a clinical effect in favor of acupuncture for MNDs, these studies scored at most 2/5 on the validated Jadad 1996 criteria for methodological quality.

A randomized, controlled trial examining standardized acupuncture needle points versus control points for neck and shoulder pain by He and colleagues[20] (2004) showed no significant effect on pain intensity until 6 to 7 treatments were completed. The investigators concluded that 8 to 10 acupuncture treatments should be given within a few weeks for relief of neck and shoulder pain. In this study, the treatment group had less intense pain than the control group at 3-year follow-up, but not at 6-month follow-up. The investigators surmised the duration of the treatment effect was probably due to breaking the patient's chronic pain cycle, rather than the acupuncture treatment effect persisting for 3 years. In addition, the lack of significant effect at 6-month follow-up may have been due to the persistence of a placebo effect on the control group at 6-months, which was not as robust at 3 years.

Acupuncture for MNDs has also been studied in comparison to nonsham controls. Coan and colleagues[21] (1982) showed that acupuncture is more effective at pain relief than a wait-list control for patients with chronic mechanical neck pain and radicular symptoms with Jadad score 3/5. Irnich and colleagues[22] (2001) showed acupuncture to be significantly better than massage for MNDs at short-term follow-up (<3 months) with Jadad score 2/5. A meta-analysis of three trials[22–24] performed by The Cochrane Collaboration showed moderate evidence (three trials, 338 participants) that acupuncture is more effective than inactive treatment for pain relief for patients with chronic MND measured at short-term follow up.[25] In the intermediate (3–12 months) and long-term follow-up categories (>12 months) in this Cochrane review, a single high-quality but underpowered study compared acupuncture with sham and showed no effect.

A cohort study by Blossfeldt[26] (2004) showed an overall success rate of 68% of acupuncture for chronic neck pain, with success defined as 50% or greater improvement of pain at the completion of three or more treatments. However, the study was not blinded, had no formal inclusion or exclusion criteria, did not include a control group, and treatments were individualized rather than standardized. Although Blossfeldt's study does not prove a treatment effect of acupuncture for chronic neck pain, it is an example of a relatively high level of self-reported patient improvement for a low-risk treatment. Of the 172 patients Blossfeldt treated, only two had complications, including one skin reaction and one migraine headache.

Acupuncture is a relatively safe modality for mechanical neck pain. A systematic review on the safety of acupuncture by Ernst and White[27] 2001 showed the most common adverse events were needle pain (1%–45%), fatigue (2%–41%), and bleeding (0.03%–38%). The incidences of syncope and feeling faint ranged from 0% to 0.3%. Pneumothorax was rare, occurring only twice in nearly a quarter of a million treatments. Overall, acupuncture for mechanical neck disorders is relatively safe. Some evidence exists that it has a beneficial clinical effect for pain relief in the short-term. Further studies are needed to clarify the possible long-term effects and to examine which treatment strategies work best for various cervical conditions.

TENS

TENS, or transcutaneous electrical nerve stimulation, is the application of a pulsed electrical current through the skin to peripheral sensory nerves for the control of pain. Muscle contractions may occur as a side effect, although they are not the primary goal as in neuromuscular electrical stimulation.[28] TENS is often applied via a portable unit consisting of a battery, signal generator, and electrodes. Currents are usually less than 100 mA with pulse rates ranging anywhere from 2 to 200 Hz. Placement of TENS electrodes is subjective, and painful sites, sites contralateral to the pain, nerves, trigger points, and even acupuncture points have been targeted.[29]

The advantages of TENS include relative comfort, rapid-onset of therapeutic effect, capability for continuous and portable use, and applicability to a variety of pain conditions. The main disadvantages are the relatively short-duration and poor carryover of the treatment effects.

Serious complications from TENS are rare. Manufacturer-listed contraindications include pregnancy, cardiac pacemaker, and epilepsy. Electrode placement over the anterior neck should be avoided, as carotid sinus stimulation could lead to vasovagal hypotension and glottic or laryngeal nerve stimulation could lead to laryngospasm and airway occlusion. Electrode placement near active malignancy should also be avoided without caution due to promotion of cell growth by electrical currents in vitro. Electrodes should be placed over healthy, normal skin due to the risk of damaging frail skin or causing burns in insensate skin. Contact dermatitis may occur, and hypoallergenic electrodes are available. Driving or operating potentially hazardous equipment should not be done during TENS.[30]

High frequency stimulation reduces pain by depolarizing type 1 afferents in muscle and skin which competes with signals from painful nerve endings per the Gate Theory of Pain. Low frequency stimulation (1 to 10 mA) is associated with the release of endorphins and serotonin.[28]

The choice of frequency may be directed by the clinical diagnosis. For example, in a randomized, double-blinded, controlled trial of 32 subjects, Walsh and colleagues[31] (1995) found that low-frequency TENS at 4 Hz was more effective in decreasing ischemically-induced pain than 110 Hz TENS, placebo, and no treatment. TENS at 2 Hz may be helpful for postoperative and radicular pain, although this intervention was not placebo-controlled.[32]

Three trials reported immediate posttreatment pain relief when using TENS for chronic cervicalgia in comparison to sham controls.[33–35] Frequencies varied from 60 to 143 Hz and schedules varied from 1 to 10 treatments. Various studies have examined the addition of TENS to other treatment modalities. Chiu and colleagues[36] (2005) compared three groups consisting of infrared irradiation, infrared irradiation plus TENS, and infrared irradiation plus exercise. When infrared irradiation was combined with either TENS or exercise, subjects showed significant improvements in disability, isometric neck muscle strength, and pain scores. However, TENS was no more effective than exercise.

In another modality-combining study by Hou and colleagues[37] (2002,) the use of TENS for cervical myofascial pain was examined. Treatment groups consisted of active range of motion exercises plus warm packs versus the former combined with TENS and either ischemic compression of myofascial trigger points or stretch and spray technique. The groups combining TENS and a myofascial release technique showed significant improvements in pain tolerance and visual analog scale pain scores.

Hendriks and Horgan[38] (1996) studied the addition of Ultra-Reiz TENS at 143 Hz to a treatment regimen of ice, physiotherapy, postural education, and cervical collar use for patients with acute whiplash-associated disorders. The addition of Ultra-Reiz TENS to the treatments resulted in significant pain intensity reduction and improved cervical range of motion at the end of a 6-week treatment regimen. However, the outcome assessor may not have been blinded.

Nordemar and Thorner[39] (1981) compared the effects of TENS, cervical collars, and manual therapy for acute cervical pain. Improvement was rapid in all groups, although TENS use led to more rapid restoration of cervical mobility. Farina and colleagues[40] (2004) examined the effect of TENS at 100 Hz compared with frequency-modulated electromagnetic stimulation from 1 to 40 Hz (FREMS) and both were shown to be similarly effective at visual analog scale pain score reduction.

In a study by Escortell and colleagues[41] (2010) patients with mechanical neck disorders were randomized to either TENS at 80 Hz or manual therapy (neuromuscular techniques, post-isometric stretching, spray and stretch, and Jones technique.) Both treatments resulted in greater than half of the patients having significantly reduced visual analog scale pain scores at short-term follow-up. Neither treatment was shown to be more effective. Success rates decreased to one-third of patients at a 6-month follow-up.

A recent Cochrane review by Kroeling and colleagues[42] (2010) summarized the evidence for TENS for neck pain. This modality might be more effective than placebo, but has not been shown to be more effective than other interventions. When assessing the included trials, funding biases and small sample sizes were considered. The quality of available evidence, as per the review authors, was low to very low. It has been noted by other investigators that proper blinding of TENS for research purposes is difficult.[43] Further research may change estimations of the effectiveness of TENS on cervical disorders.

MASSAGE THERAPY

Massage is one of the oldest healing arts. Chinese records dating back 3,000 years document its use; the ancient Hindus, Persians, and Egyptians applied forms of massage for many ailments; and Hippocrates wrote papers recommending the use of rubbing and friction for joint and circulatory problems.[44] Goals of massage are to restore the patient to optimal function, help prevent future injury, promote better posture, and create more efficient use of muscle activation.

The most commonly involved tissues in a patient with neck pain are the sternocleidomastoids, scalenes, upper trapezius, levator scapulas, splenius capitis, pectoralis, and intercostals as well as the surrounding fascia. Excessive tension in any or all of these tissues, bilaterally or unilaterally, can produce mild-to-severe discomfort, compromise natural mobility, create pathologic cervical vertebral alignment, and can activate headaches.[45,46]

Massage techniques are too numerous to describe in specific detail for scope of this article, but most fall under one or more of the categories of: "effleurage" or gliding; "petrissage" or kneading; "tappotement" or tapping; and friction, including static pressure, myofascial release, cross fibril, and vibration. All of these techniques elicit mechanical compression and stimulation to soft tissue.[47]

Massage therapy has been shown to have direct benefits, including improved circulation, cumulative rise in oxytocin, decrease in basal hypothalamic-pituitary axis activity, enhanced feelings of relaxation, increased feelings of well-being, and reduction in measures of anxiety, depression, and pain.[48,49] Massage also has been shown to increase serotonin levels and promote reduction of analgesic use.[45]

Chen and Grinnel[50] (1995) found that stretching skeletal muscle in the physiologic range more than doubled the spontaneous release of acetylcholine from its motor nerve terminal. This raises end-plate potentials, which causes activation of integrins in the cytoplasmic membrane and an increase the activation of calcium. Thus, massage, particularly myofascial techniques, may improve muscular performance and tone.

Massage has the added benefit of increasing blood and lymphatic fluid flow. Studies have shown that mechanical energy is able to stimulate new capillary formation of arterial, venous, and lymphatic vessels.[51,52] These also showed that smooth muscle cells significantly increased production of collagen after the application of mechanical stimuli. In addition, mechanical signals (ie, produced by static friction or pressure incorporated in massage) are able to augment cell proliferation (especially fibroblasts), stimulating the healing process at the site of injury.[53] As a result of the mechanical effect of massage strokes, more blood is pushed through the massaged area. As such, massage strokes support the venous and lymphatic drainage from the massaged area.[47]

Survey studies document that recipients of massage have improved joint mobility and pain reduction.[54] For this reason, some institutions have integrated massage into patient care programs. A study of 24 hospitalized patients with neck pain at the University of South Carolina found that pain scores were significantly reduced immediately following therapeutic massage.[55,56]

A combination of massage techniques applied to the cervical, shoulder, and upper back musculature can increase cervical active and passive ranges of motion, reduce reported headache severity, and reduce pain complaints. These changes can often be achieved in a few sessions. To be most effective, massage treatment should be followed up by patient education regarding proper diaphragmatic breathing techniques for relaxation, cervical stretches to maintain the length relationships achieved by the massage, as well as strengthening exercises for the muscles of the cervical spine. Contraindications to massage include cancer, unstable fractures, severe hypertension, fever, contagious skin condition, and tumors.

YOGA

Yoga is a popular mind-body exercise that couples physical exercise with mental focus through breathing and meditation. There has been a dramatic increase in the popularity of yoga in America over the last decade. In 1998, a United States national survey estimated that 15.0 million American adults used yoga at least once in their lifetime and 7.5 million during the previous year. Participators reported using yoga for both wellness and health issues; specifically, 21% of respondents used yoga in the previous 12 months for back or neck pain.[57] More recently, according to Yoga Research and Education Council statistics, 15 million Americans practiced yoga more than three times weekly in 2003.[58]

Although there are no published studies on the effectiveness of yoga for neck pain, there are several studies focusing on the role of yoga in managing chronic low back pain (CLBP). In 2005, Williams and colleagues[59] evaluated the efficacy of a yoga intervention compared with an educational control group on pain-related outcomes in patients with CLBP. They showed that yoga could significantly reduce pain and disability and decrease use of pain medications in CLBP patients. Sherman and colleagues[60] conducted a randomized controlled trial in 2005 comparing the effect of yoga classes to conventional exercise classes and a self-care book in patients with CLBP. They concluded that yoga was more effective in reducing pain and improving functional status than a self-care book. More recently, in 2009 Williams and colleagues[61] published another study on the effectiveness and efficacy of yoga for CLBP compared with standard medical care. They found that yoga reduced pain intensity and functional disability in patients with CLBP; there was also a trend in the yoga group to reduced pain medication usage.

There are also several studies on the effect of yoga on stress, anxiety, and depression. A pilot study by Woolery and colleagues[62] in 2004 found a yoga program to be beneficial on psychological outcomes in mildly depressed patients. Michalsen and colleagues[63] reported that a yoga program markedly alleviated perceived stress and related anxiety and depression symptoms in distressed women. Interestingly, the effect of yoga on mood may be immediate. West and colleagues[64] found a single 90-minute yoga class reduced perceived stress and negative mood directly after the yoga practice in healthy subjects.

It follows that yoga may have similar benefits for patients with neck pain. Patients with chronic neck pain may have associated biomechanical deficits, including poor posture, contracted upper neck muscles, and weak scapular stabilizers. With chronic neck pain, there may also be associated symptoms of stress, anxiety, or depression. Because of yoga's physical emphasis on postural restoration, flexibility, and strengthening; and mental emphasis on relaxation and meditation; it may reduce pain, improve function, and lower stress, anxiety, and depression in patients with chronic neck pain.

Physically, yoga focuses on improving patient posture, flexibility, and strength. One of the goals of the asanas, or postures, is to re-establish a normal cervical curve or neutral cervical spine. One achieves this by cultivating a conscious awareness of alignment throughout the yoga practice, during all standing and sitting poses. Another focus of the asanas is to improve flexibility. In some instances, upper neck muscles, including the upper trapezius and levator scapulae, can assume a state of constant isometric contraction against the weight of the head and downward pull of gravity. The anterior chest muscles such as the pectoralis also become contracted. The focus of several asanas is to bring awareness to the upper trapezius and levator scapulae, and attempt to reduce unconscious contraction of these muscles. For the pectoralis muscles, many asanas focus on lifting and opening up the chest. After flexibility is achieved in the tight muscles, focus shifts to strengthening weak muscles. In chronic neck pain, the lower trapezius and rhomboids, important stabilizers of the spine, can become weak. Several poses activate scapular stabilizers, lower trapezius, and rhomboids.

In addition to the physical focus on posture, flexibility, and strength, yoga's mental focus through breathing and meditation targets stress and anxiety. Pranayama, the breathing technique used with asana, can be a powerful way to relax and is considered by many to be the first step toward relieving neck tension. Meditation has also been shown to be effective in managing chronic pain. Kabat-Zinn[65] studied 51 chronic pain patients, including those with low back, headache, neck, and shoulder pain, in a preliminary cohort study. A 10-week stress reduction and relaxation program taught patients hatha yoga, emphasizing mindfulness, self-regulation, meditation, and detached observation, which theoretically "uncouples" the sensory experience from the "affective alarm reaction." At 10 weeks, 50% of subjects had pain score reductions of greater than or equal to 50%. A follow up study of 12 cycles of classes over a 4-year period totaling 225 subjects was later conducted by Kabat-Zinn and colleagues.[66] These subjects engaged in the same methods of stress reduction described in his preliminary work. When questionnaires were given to these groups of cohorts, 60% to 72% of subjects rated their pain as "moderate" or "great improvement" and 30% to 55% rated their pain as "greatly improved." Only 1% to 15% rated their pain as worse and 25% rated their pain as the same. Eighty-six percent reported that they gained something of lasting value or importance. Of the subjects, 115 reported free comments in questionnaire. Of these, 20% reported a "new outlook on life" and

40% reported ability to control, understand, or cope better with pain and stress. At 4 years, 81% of respondents reported that they still meditated. Depending on follow-up interval of these cohorts, 40% to 70% of responders reported that they still practiced yoga. Rosenswaig and colleagues[67] recently investigated effects on 133 subjects who underwent 8 weeks of mindfulness training, focusing on meditation techniques, including body scan, awareness of breathing, awareness of emotions, mindful yoga and walking, mindful eating, and mindful listening. Subjects with back or neck pain (n = 35) showed significant improvement on six of eight Medical Outcomes Study 36-Item Short-Form Health Survey (SF-36) indices, including bodily pain.

Patients with a recent injury such as a motor vehicle collision or fall; radicular pain in the arms or legs; neurologic symptoms such as paresthesias, weakness, or gait instability; persistent or recurrent pain; or dizziness and nausea should seek medical evaluation and clearance before starting a yoga practice. Also, some poses should be avoided in patients with neck pain as they can strain the neck and lead to serious injury. In the absence of these contraindications, yoga can be helpful in diminishing pain, improving function, and reducing stress and anxiety in patients with neck pain. As with many modalities, more well controlled randomized studies are needed to further evaluate the role of yoga in managing neck pain.

TAI CHI CHUAN

Tai chi chuan (tai chi) is an ancient Chinese martial art that focuses on slow, controlled, continuous movements coordinated with breathing, resulting in motion meditation.[68] The swaying movement of Tai Chi demands more range of motion and its slow speed creates less impact forces than walking. Modern styles of tai chi trace their development to the five traditional schools: Chen, Yang, Hao, Wu, and Sun. Traditional Chinese medicine theorizes that disease results when the flow of Qi (internal energy) is blocked and when there is disharmony between yin and yang forces. Tai chi can balance these forces along with improving function through movement and medication. Most research is conducted on the Sun and Yang styles, although many research studies do not mention the style of tai chi in their intervention.[69] The Sun style is currently endorsed by the US Arthritis Foundation as low impact exercise that can reduce joint pain.[70]

Between 1974 and 2010, approximately 475 English studies on the benefits of tai chi were published; 20% of these were randomly controlled trials.[71] Overall, these studies show some physical and psychological benefits. Unfortunately, most studies compare tai chi to no other intervention, and there are no direct studies on tai chi and neck pain. The strongest proven benefit of tai chi is improved balance and fall reduction, which can prevent exacerbations of neck pain and may improve head-down posture, commonly observed in those fearful of falling.[72] Chen also found that tai chi practice was associated with less fear of falling, increased confidence in balance and movement, increased overall well-being, and improved body stability.[73] Some studies state that tai chi may improve sleep, decrease tension, reduce anger, and improve self-esteem, but likely not more than other interventions that include meditation.[74,75] A 15-week intervention of tai chi practice was effective in reducing the impact of life on tension headaches.[76] Several of these studies showed better posture stability in the elderly and improved posture in young adults. One study of 56 people measured range of motion and found a lessening of "poking chin," head tilting, and shoulders level.[77] A longitudinal study found people who practice tai chi for years had better eye-hand coordination with fewer submovements when attempting a task.[78] Tai chi has been shown to increase general function in specific diseases of osteoarthritis,[69,79] rheumatoid arthritis,[71] and ankylosing spondylitis.[80]

Although tai chi has not been shown to worsen any disease process with tender swollen joints,[71] research suggests that there is no benefit in joint disease modification. In addition, it has not been shown to increase strength or flexibility of the upper extremities.[79]

Tai chi has a significantly higher level of participation than physical therapy. This can be attributed to the benefits of group therapy, having a mind-body intervention,[75] and being more appealing than range of motion exercises.[71] Tai chi also has the benefit of being considered safer than most forms of exercise,[69] although studies do report individuals dropping out due to knee or back pain.[72] In one small study, 14% of tai chi students (or 2 people out of 14) had injuries compared with 30% of those practicing karate. Training greater than 3 hours per week was also a significant predictor of injury.[81]

Although there are no studies specifically on the use of tai chi for neck pain, this modality may benefit patients when neck pain is associated with poor neck posture and stress. Tai chi's mind-body component might help it be a more effective and satisfying intervention than physical therapy, and it is safe to recommend to even frail patients.[71] Future studies need to be done to better understand the association of tai chi with neck pain and functional outcomes.

FELDENKRAIS

The Feldenkrais Method of somatic education offers a clinical tool to help alleviate neck pain and to restore natural function. A practice of neuromuscular re-education that allows a person to sense their whole self more clearly, Feldenkrais may be used for headaches, cervicalgia, postlaminectomy symptoms, degenerative disc disease, thoracic outlet syndrome, postural malalignment, hyperlordosis, and flat cervical spine.

This modality is named after its founder, Moshe Feldenkrais DSc (1904–1984), and consists of two trademark lesson plans: Awareness Through Movement (ATM) and Functional Integration. ATM lessons can be taught in a group setting where a practitioner verbally guides the patients through a sequence of gentle, pain-free movements with the goal of becoming more deeply aware of their own biomechanics.

Functional Integration lessons are individualized sessions where the practitioner communicates through gentle touch, guided movements, and verbal cueing, to lead the patient toward sensing tension and patterns that contribute to deficient functioning. The patient stays fully clothed and is always an active participant in the healing process. The learning process is facilitated by moving in pain-free ranges, thus avoiding sympathetic arousal that could exacerbate symptoms.[82,83] The intended outcome of Feldenkrais lessons is that the patient moves with increased fluidity, greater active range of motion without increased effort, decreased pain, and an improved sense of well-being.

The Feldenkrais principle of maximum efficiency with minimal effort allows a patient to learn through experience and sensation, to function with less joint strain, less biomechanical error, and decrease the kinematic wear and tear on joints that shows up as dysfunction.[84,85]

From the Feldenkrais perspective, guiding a patient with neck pain toward relief and recovery often requires looking beyond the cervical spine. Within this perspective, cervical pain can be literally originating from the neck, but could also be initiated from any number of other sources. These include insufficient breathing patterns, pelvic obliquities, insufficient differentiation of the eye or head movements, overuse of upper extremity musculature, restricted lumbar motion, or even a foot injury that causes malfunctioning up the skeletal chain. The practitioner observes the global movement of a patient with neck complaints, then attempts to unravel any limitations of movement so that the original neck pain is diffused and function improves.

In a randomized control trial comparing physiotherapy and the Feldenkrais method in a control group in female industrial workers with neck and shoulder pain, Lundblad and colleagues[86] found that the Feldenkrais group showed significant decreases in neck and shoulder complaints and in disability during leisure time. The two other groups showed no change (physiotherapy group) or worsening of complaints (control group).

The efficacy and cost of using group Feldenkrais lessons with chronic pain patients was studied by Bearman and Shafarman.[87] Medicaid recipients with chronic headaches and/or musculoskeletal problems reported more mobility and decreased perception of pain, both immediately after the program and in a 1-year follow-up questionnaire, using the National Pain Data Bank protocol of the American Academy of Pain Management. Patient costs dropped from an average of $141 per month to $82 per month, representing a 40% savings.[87]

Quantifying the goal of achieving functional movement with less effort and greater efficiency was studied by Brown and Kegerris.[88] This small study used 21 subjects, divided into two groups, to measure the muscular activation during an ATM class by use of electromyographic biofeedback equipment. It also recorded subjects' perceptual recognition of changes and whether such perceived changes were due to use of suggestion, imagery, and visualization. Both groups received the same 45 minute lesson; one listened to the lesson in its entirety, while the other received an edited version where all references to imagery, visualization, or cues pertaining to lightness, comfort, or ease were removed. Both groups showed a decrease in electromyographic activity and in perceived exertion. Although not compared with any control groups, the experimenters concluded, "This study supports the use of Feldenkrais Method clinically for increasing attention to posturing, movements, and changes in muscular activity."[88]

In another study by Kerr and colleagues[89] (2002), the State-Trait Anxiety Inventory[90,91] was administered to volunteers at the beginning and end of the first, fifth, and tenth (final) 1-hour ATM lesson. Although there was no control, an overall significant decrease in anxiety scores was measured. Although many subjective reports of improvements in quality of movement and pain relief from the Feldenkrais method exist, future clinical studies using standardized outcome tools are needed to help objectify these improvements.

SUMMARY

Of the multitude of treatment options for the management of neck pain, no obvious single treatment modality has been shown to be most efficacious. As such, the clinician should consider alternative treatment modalities if a modality is engaging, available, financially feasible, potentially efficacious, and is low risk for the patient. As evidence-based medicine for neck pain develops, the clinician is faced with the challenge of which treatments to encourage patients to pursue. Treatment modalities explored in this article, including chiropractic, acupuncture, TENS, massage, yoga, tai chi, and Feldenkrais, represent reasonable CAM methods to offer patients with neck pain.

REFERENCES

1. McPhee SJ, Papadakis MA, Tierney LM, editors. Current medical diagnosis and treatment. 46th edition. New York: McGraw-Hill; 2007.

2. Barnes PM, Bloom B, Nahin RL. Complementary and alternative medicine use among adults and children: United States, 2007. National health statistics reports. vol. 12. Hyattsville (MD): Centers for Disease Control and Prevention, National Center for Health Statistics; 2008.
3. Eisenberg DM, Davis RB, Ettner SL, et al. Trends in alternative medicine use in the United States, 1990–1997: results of a follow-up national survey. JAMA 1998;280(18):1569–75.
4. Liebenson C. Rehabilitation of the spine. A practitioner's manual. Philadelphia: Lippincott Williams & Wilkins; 2007. p. 3–29; 72–90; 487–509; 753–75; 852–85.
5. Triano JJ. Biomechanics of spinal manipulative therapy. Spine 2001;1(2):121–30.
6. Shekelle PG. Spinal manipulation. Spine 1994;19:858–61.
7. Gross AR, Hoving JL, Haines TA, et al. Cervical overview group. A Cochrane review of manipulation and mobilization for mechanical neck disorders. Spine 2004;29:1541–8.
8. Miller J, Gross A, D'Sylva J, et al. Manual therapy and exercise for neck pain: a systematic review. Man Ther 2010;15:334–54.
9. Hurwitz EL, Carragee EJ, Velde van der G, et al. Treatment of neck pain: noninvasive interventions. Results of the Bone and Joint Decade 2000–2010 task force on neck pain and its associated disorders. Spine 2008;33:S123–52.
10. Gross A, Miller J, D'Sylva J, et al. Manipulation or mobilization for neck pain: a Cochrane review. Man Ther 2010;15:315–33.
11. Cleland JA, Childs JD, McRae M, et al. Immediate effects of thoracic manipulation in patients with neck pain: a randomized clinical trial. Man Ther 2005;10:127–35.
12. Norlander S, Nordgren B. Clinical symptoms related to pain and mobility in the cervicothoracic spine. Scand J Rehabil Med 1998;30:243–51.
13. Cleland JA, Glynn P, Whitman JM, et al. Short-term effects of thrust versus non-thrust mobilization/manipulation directed at the thoracic spine in patients with neck pain: a randomized clinical trial. Phys Ther 2007;87:431–40.
14. Senstad O, Leboeuf-Yde C, Borchgrevink C. Frequency and characteristics of side effects of spinal manipulative therapy. Spine 1997;22:435–40.
15. Michaeli A. Reported occurrence and nature of complications following manipulative physiotherapy in South Africa. Aust J Physiother 1993;39:309–15.
16. Haldeman S, Kolbeck FJ, McGregor M. Stroke, cerebral artery dissection, and cervical spine manipulation therapy. J Neurol 2002;249:1098–104.
17. Cassidy JD, Boyle E, Cote P, et al. Risk of vertebrobasilar stroke and chiropractic care: results of a population-based case-control and case-crossover study. Spine 2008;33:S176–83.
18. Birch S, Jamison R. Controlled trial of Japanese acupuncture for chronic myofascial neck pain: assessment of specific and nonspecific effects of treatment. Clin J Pain 1998;14:248–55.
19. White PF, Craig WF, Vakharia AS, et al. Percutaneous neuromodulation therapy: does the location of electrical stimulation effect the acute analgesic response? Anesth Analg 2000;91:949–54.
20. He D, Veiersted KB, Hostmark AT, et al. Effect of acupuncture treatment on chronic neck and shoulder pain in sedentary female workers: a 6-month and 3-year follow-up study. Pain 2004;109:299–307.
21. Coan RM, Wong G, Coan PL. The acupuncture treatment of neck pain: a randomized controlled study. Am J Chin Med 1982;9(4):326–32.
22. Irnich D, Behrens N, Molzen H, et al. Randomized trial of acupuncture compared with conventional massage and "sham" laser acupuncture for treatment of chronic neck pain. BMJ 2001;322:1574–8.

23. Vickers AJ. Statistical re-analysis of four recent randomized trials of acupuncture for pain using analysis of covariance. Clin J Pain 2004;20(5):319–23.

24. White P, Lewith G, Prescott P, et al. Acupuncture versus placebo for the treatment of chronic mechanical neck pain. Ann Intern Med 2004;141:920–8.

25. Trinh K, Graham N, Gross A; Cervical Overview Group, et al. Acupuncture for neck disorders. Cochrane Database Syst Rev 2010;3:CD004870.

26. Blossfeldt P. Acupuncture for chronic neck pain—a cohort study in an NHS pain clinic. Acupunct Med 2004;22:146–51.

27. Ernst E, White AR. Prospective studies of the safety of acupuncture: a systematic review. Am J Med 2001;110:481–5.

28. Pape KE, Chipman ML. Electrotherapy in rehabilitation. In: DeLisa JA, editor. Physical Medicine and Rehabilitation, Principles and Practice. Philadelphia: Lippincott Williams and Wilkins; 2005. p. 435–7.

29. Basford JR. Therapeutic physical agents. In: DeLisa JA, editor. Physical Medicine and Rehabilitation, Principles and Practice. Philadelphia: Lippincott Williams and Wilkins; 2005. p. 262–3.

30. Johnson MI. Transcutaneous electrical nerve stimulation (TENS). In: Watson T, editor. Electrotherapy: evidence-based practice. Twelfth edition. Philadelphia: Elsevier; 2008. p. 264–7.

31. Walsh D, Liggett C, Baxter D, et al. A double-blind investigation of the hypoalgesic effects of transcutaneous electrical nerve stimulation upon experimentally induced ischaemic pain. Pain 1995;61(1):39–45.

32. Carrol E, Badura A. Focal intense brief transcutaneous electric nerve stimulation for treatment of radicular and postthoracotomy pain. Arch Phys Med Rehabil 2001;82:262–4.

33. Hsueh TC, Cheng PT, Kuan TS, et al. The immediate effectiveness of electrical nerve stimulation and electrical muscle stimulation on myofascial trigger points. Am J Phys Med Rehabil 1997;76:471–6.

34. Smania N, Corato E, Fiaschi A, et al. Repetitive magnetic stimulation: a novel therapeutic approach for myofascial pain syndrome. J Neurol 2005;252:307–14.

35. Flynn T. A comparative study between ultrareiz and ultrasound in the treatment for relief of pain in whiplash injuries. Physiotherapy Ireland 1987;8(1):11–4.

36. Chiu TW, Hui-Chan C, Cheing G. A randomized clinical trial of TENS and exercise for patients with chronic neck pain. Clin Rehabil 2005;19:850–60.

37. Hou CR, Tsai LC, Cheng KF, et al. Immediate effects of various physical therapeutic modalities on cervical myofascial pain and trigger point sensitivity. Arch Phys Med Rehabil 2002;83:1406–14.

38. Hendriks O, Horgan A. Ultra-reiz current as an adjunct to standard physiotherapy treatment of the acute whiplash patient. Physiotherapy Ireland 1996; 17(1):13–7.

39. Nordemar R, Thorner C. Treatment of acute cervical pain: a comparative group study. Pain 1981;10:93–101.

40. Farina S, Casarotto M, Benelle M, et al. A randomized controlled study on the effect of two different treatments in myofascial pain syndrome. Eur Medicophys 2004;40:293–301.

41. Escortell-Mayor E, Riesgo-Fuertes R, Garrido-Elustondo S, et al; TEMA-TENS Group. Primary care randomized clinical trial: manual therapy effectiveness in comparison with TENS in patients with neck pain. Man Ther 2011;16(1): 66–73.

42. Kroeling P, Gross A, Goldsmith CH, et al. Electrotherapy for neck pain. Cochrane Library 2010;3:1–71.

43. Deyo RA, Walsh NE, Martin DC, et al. A controlled trial of transcutaneous electrical nerve stimulation and exercise for chronic low back pain. N Engl J Med 1990; 322(23):1627–34.
44. Clavert RN. the history of massage: an illustrated survey from around the world. Babylonia, Egypt, China, India: Healing Press; 2002.
45. Hernandez-Reif M, Field T, Dieter J, et al. Migraine headaches are reduced by massage therapy. Int J Neurosci 1998;96:1–11.
46. Quinn C, Chandler C, Moraska A. Massage therapy and frequency of chronic tension headaches. Am J Public Health 2002;92:1657–61.
47. Turchaninov R. Research and Massage Therapy, Part 1: The science to back it up. Available at: http://www.massagetherapy.com/articles/index.php/article_id/333/Research–Massage-Therapy-Part-1. Accessed April 26, 2011.
48. Binesh N, Cohen RM, Moser FG, et al. Does Massage Therapy affect Brain Metabolites? Int J Alter Med 2008;5(2). Available at: http://www.ispub.com/journal/the_internet_journal_of_alternative_medicine/volume_5_number_2_3/article/does_massage_therapy_affect_brain_metabolites.html. Accessed April 23, 2011.
49. Sharpe PA, Williams HG, Granner ML, et al. A randomised study of the effects of massage therapy compared to guided relaxation on well-being and stress perception among older adults. Complement Ther Med 2007;15(3):157–63.
50. Chen BM, Grinnell AD. Integrins and modulation of transmitter release from motor nerve terminals by stretch. Science 1995;269:1578–80.
51. Shirinsky VP, Antonov AS, Birukov KG, et al. Mechano-chemical control of human endothelium orientation and size. J Cell Biol 1989;109:331–9.
52. Leung DYM, Gladov S, Mathews MB. Cyclic stretching stimulates synthesis of martix components by arterial smooth muscle in vitro. Science 1976;191:475–7.
53. Curtis ASG, Sheehar GM. The control of cell division by tension or diffusion. Nature 1978;274:52–3.
54. Anderson PG, Cutshall SM. Massage therapy and comfort intervention for cardiac surgery patients. Clin Nurse Spec 2007;21(3):161–7.
55. Ferner TE, Plewa MC. Poster session abstracts: massage therapy effectively reduces pain in hospitalized patients. Cincinnati (OH): AMTA national convention; 2007.
56. Verhagen AP, Karels C, Bierma-Zeinstra SM, et al. Ergonomic and physiotherapeutic interventions for treating work-related complaints of the arms, neck, or shoulders in adults. Cochrane Database Syst Rev 2006;3:CD003471.
57. Saper RB, Eiseberg DM, Davis RB, et al. Prevalence and patterns of adult yoga use in the United States: results of a national survey. Altern Ther Health Med 2004;10:1–9.
58. Jacobs BP, Mehling W, Goldberg HA, et al. Feasibility of conducting a clinical trial on Hatha yoga for chronic low back pain: methodological lessons. Altern Ther Health Med 2004;10:80–3.
59. Williams K, Steinberg L, Petronis J. Therapeutic application of Iyengar yoga for healing chronic low back pain. Int J Yoga Ther 2003;13:55–67.
60. Sherman KJ, Cherkin DC, Erro J, et al. Comparing yoga, exercise, and a self-care book for chronic low back pain: a randomized, controlled trial. Ann Intern Med 2005;143:849–56.
61. Williams J, Abilds C, Steinberg L. Evaluation of the effectiveness and efficacy of Iyengar yoga therapy on chronic low back pain. Spine 2009;34(19):2066–76.
62. Woolery A, Myers H, Sternlieb B, et al. A yoga intervention for young adults with elevated symptoms of depression. Altern Ther Health Med 2004;10:60–3.

63. Michalsen A, Grossman P, Acil A. Rapid stress reduction and anxiolysis among distressed women as a consequence of a three-month intensive yoga program. Med Sci Monit 2005;11(12):555–61.
64. West J, Otte C, Geher K. Effects of Hatha yoga and African dance on perceived stress, affect, and salivary cortisol. Ann Behav Med 2004;28:114–8.
65. Kabat-Zinn J. An outpatient program in behavioral medicine for chronic pain patients based on the practice of mindfulness meditation: theoretical considerations and preliminary results. Gen Hosp Psychiatry 1982;4:33–47.
66. Kabat-Zinn J, Lipwort L, Burney R, et al. Four-year follow-up of a meditation-based program for the self-regulation of chronic pain: treatment outcomes and compliance. Clin J Pain 1987;2:159–73.
67. Rosenswaig S, Greeson JM, Reibel DK, et al. Mindfulness-based stress reduction for chronic pain conditions: variation in treatment outcomes and role of home meditation practice. J Psychosom Res 2010;68:29–36.
68. Wayne P, Kaptuchuk T. Challenges inherent to t'ai chi research: part 1—t'ai chi as a complex multicomponent intervention. J Altern Complement Med 2008;14(1): 95–102.
69. Hall A, Maher C. The effectiveness of Tai Chi for chronic musculoskeletal pain conditions: a systemic review and meta-analysis. Arthritis Rheum 2009;61: 717–24.
70. Available at: http://www.arthritis.org/tai-chi.php. Accessed April 11, 2010.
71. Yeh G. Commentary on the Cochrane review of Tai Chi for rheumatoid arthritis. Explorer 2008;4(4):275–7.
72. Wolf S, Sattin R. Intense tai chi exercise training and fall occurrences in older, transitionally frail adults: a randomized, controlled trial. J Am Geriatr Soc 2003; 51(12):1693–701.
73. Chen KM, Snyder M. Research-based use of Tai Chi/movement therapy as a nursing intervention. J Holist Nurs 1999;17:267.
74. Wang WC, Zhang AL, Rasmussen B, et al. The effect of Tai chi on psychosocial well-being: a systematic review of random controlled trials. J Acupunct Meridian Stud 2009;2(3):171–81.
75. Wahbeh H, Elsas SM, Oken BS. Mind-body interventions: applications in neurology. Neurology 2008;70(24):2321–8.
76. Abbott RB, Hui KK, Hays RD, et al. A randomized controlled trial of Tai Chi for tension headaches. Evid Based Complement Alternat Med 2007;4(1):107–13.
77. Gao KL, Tsang WW. Effects of short term tai training on spinal posture of young university students presented at the XXIth Congress of the International Society of Biomechanics. Taipei, Taiwan, July 5. J Biomech 2007;40(Suppl 2):S04.
78. Pei YC, Chou SW. Eye hand coordination of elderly people who practice Tai Chi Chuan. J Formos Med Assoc 2008;107(2):103–10.
79. Song R, Lee E. Effects of tai chi exercise on pain, balance, muscle strength, and perceived difficulties in physical functioning in older women with osteoarthritis: a randomized clinical trial. J Rheumatol 2003;30(9):2039–44.
80. Lee EN, Kim YH, Chung WT, et al. Tai chi for disease activity and flexibility in patients with ankylosing spondylitis—a controlled clinical trial. Evid Based Complement Alternat Med 2008;5(4):457–62.
81. Zetaruk MN, Violan MA. Injuries in martial arts: a comparison of five styles. Br J Sports Med 2005;39(1):29–33.
82. Syrjala KL, Yi JC. Relaxation and imagery techniques. In: Ballantyne JC, Fishman SM, Rathmell JP, editors. Bonica's Management of Pain. 4 edition. Philadelphia: Lippincott Williams and Wilkins; 2005. p. 1255–6.

83. Feldenkrais M. Awareness Through Movement. New York: HarperCollins; 1972. p. 91–6.
84. Hannon JC. The physics of Feldenkrais: part 5: unstable equilibrium and its application to movement therapy. J Bodywork Mov Ther 2001;5(3):207–21.
85. Feldenkrais M. Awareness Through Movement. New York: HarperCollins; 1972. p. 58.
86. Lundblad I, Elert J, Gerdle B. Randomized controlled trial of physiotherapy and Feldenkrais interventions in female workers with neck-shoulder complaints. J Occup Rehabil 1999;9(3):179–94.
87. Bearman D, Shafarman S. Feldenkrais method in the treatment of chronic pain: a study of efficacy and cost effectiveness. AJPM 1999;9(1):22–7.
88. Brown E, Kegerris S. Electromyographic activity of trunk musculature during a Feldenkrais Awareness Through Movement lesson. Isokinet Exerc Sci 1991; 1(4):216–21.
89. Kerr GA, Kotynia F, Kolt GS. Feldenkrais awareness through movement and state anxiety. J Bodywork Mov Ther 2002;6(2):102–7.
90. Spielberger C. Encyclopedia of psychology. 2010.
91. Linton SJ. A review of psychological risk factors in back and neck pain. Spine 2000;25(9):1148–56.

Interventional Procedures for Cervical Pain

Ai Mukai, MD[a],*, Vishal Kancherla, DO[b]

KEYWORDS

- Cervical • Pain • Radiculopathy • Intervention

Percutaneous interventional spinal procedures have become ubiquitous in the management of cervical pain syndromes. This article reviews the indications, contraindications, patient selection, and potential complications of epidural injections, zygapophyseal joint and medial branch nerve injections, spinal cord stimulation, and radiofrequency neurotomy. When considering interventional treatment options for cervical pain, several general principles apply. First, a systematic approach should be used to take a focused history and perform a thorough physiatric physical examination of the musculoskeletal and neurologic systems. Second, imaging studies may be used to further delineate the cause of pain. Patients should then be educated about possible diagnoses and counseled on all treatment options, including noninterventional modalities, such as physical therapy and medications. This discussion should generate a treatment plan that incorporates patient input and physician recommendations. Interventional procedures may or may not be a part of such plan. Contraindications to procedures include local infection in the area of the planned procedure, systemic infection, thrombocytopenia and other coagulopathies, pregnancy (because of need for fluoroscopic guidance), and medical instability requiring immediate medical intervention. Physiatric history and physical examination, epidemiology, surgical options, alternative and complementary treatment options, and a review of cervical spine anatomy are covered elsewhere in this issue.

After the decision is made to pursue percutaneous interventional procedures, patients must be counseled on potential risks and benefits as well as alternatives. Patients' medication lists should be reviewed to identify medications that may need to be held before a procedure. Most guidelines recommend holding anticoagulants for 3 to 5 days before a procedure.[1] Non-neuroaxial procedures may allow for more flexibility. There is controversy surrounding the use of nonsteroidal antiinflammatory

The authors have nothing to disclose.

[a] Texas Orthopedics Sports and Rehabilitation, 4700 Seton Center Parkway, Suite 200, Austin, TX 78759, USA

[b] Austin Diagnostic Clinic, 12221 North Mopac Expressway, Austin, TX 78758, USA

* Corresponding author.

E-mail address: amukai@txortho.com

drugs, aspirin, and diabetic medications before a procedure. It may be prudent to have a discussion with the clinician prescribing said medications about the potential risks of holding the medication. Patients with hypertension and diabetes should be counseled on the effect of systemic corticosteroids if the procedure involves the use of such agents. Patients with poor renal function, hepatic pathology, or any other complicated medical comorbidities may need laboratory work completed before the procedure to rule out conditions, such as thrombocytopenia or infection. Finally, the patient allergy list should be reviewed to ensure that no contraindications exist and no modifications are needed.

The physician performing the procedure also needs to be prepared for potential complications and side effects. More common immediate complications and side effects include reactions to injectates, prolonged paresthesia or motor block, increased pain, and vasovagal response. There is also rare but potentially devastating risk of dural puncture, direct trauma to a neural structure, pneumocephalus, ischemia resulting in spinal cord or brain infarction, intravascular anesthesia resulting in loss of consciousness and apnea, neuropathic reactions to the corticosteroid agent injected, epidural granuloma, and pneumothorax.[2] Subacute complications and reactions include infections, hematoma, postdural puncture headache, and possible delayed ischemia resulting in stroke. Early recognition of symptoms and preparation for immediate response can decrease the risk to patients. The use of sedation can influence the risks of the procedure, both favorably by reducing patient movement and anxiety, and adversely if patients are oversedated. Oversedation may cause inability to respond to painful stimuli, and possible respiratory and cardiovascular depression.

Radiographic guidance is routinely used in interventional procedures for the cervical spine. Care must be taken to reduce radiation risk to patients and the practitioner. Proper shielding, use of foot pedals and extension tubing, routine maintenance of equipment, reducing field of exposure through collimation, reducing time of exposure through pulsed imaging, minimizing the use of lateral visualization, and lowering the image intensifier closer to patients can all decrease radiation exposure to both patients and personnel.

CERVICAL EPIDURAL INTERVENTIONS

Cervical epidural injections are used to treat radicular pain in the cervical spine. One study shows that older patients and those with radicular pain as opposed to axial pain alone seem to benefit the most from cervical epidural steroid injections, which is similar to literature in the lumbar spine.[3] One theory behind the mechanism of action of injections is that corticosteroids interrupt the inflammatory cascade and thus reduce pain. Some research also shows that corticosteroids may block nociceptor C-fiber conduction, increase microcirculation around ischemic areas, and modulate pain transmission in the dorsal horn.[4,5]

There are 2 approaches to the cervical epidural space: interlaminar and transforaminal (**Figs. 1** and **2**). Unlike the lumbar spine, there is a paucity of research showing relative efficacy of one approach versus another or efficacy for radicular pain versus axial pain. One prospective independent clinical review showed 93% of patients with good relief of pain up to 7 months (interlaminar approach) and 2 retrospective analyses showed 60% of patients had good relief up to 6 months (selective nerve root blocks) and 20.7 months (transforaminal approach).[6–8] The most recent systematic review of the effectiveness of cervical epidural steroid injections showed significant effectiveness of epidural injections in the treatment of chronic cervical pain.[9] Although many practitioners perform a series of 3 injections 2 weeks apart, there is no evidence or consensus supporting this practice.

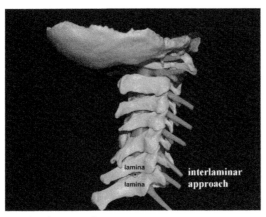

Fig. 1. Interlaminar epidural approach.

Interlaminar Cervical Epidural Injections

The interlaminar approach reaches the posterior epidural space through the interspinous ligament and the ligamentum flavum. Usually, this approach is done via a paramedian approach starting just lateral to the spinous process and directing toward midline while staying paramedian.[10] Although interlaminar injections can be performed without radiographic guidance using only the loss of resistance technique, this blind approach has been found to have a miss rate of 53%.[11] There have also been studies that showed that intravascular injections can occur in 8.5% to as high as 19.4% of injections despite no aspiration of blood and with increased incidence in patients greater than 50 years old.[12–14] Furthermore, anatomic studies have found that in almost half of the specimens studied, the ligamentum flavum did not fuse in the midline and the interspinous ligament was not present. These anatomic considerations indicate potentially higher risk of dural puncture, spinal cord injury, and misplacement of medication when radiographic guidance is not used. The cervical epidural space also narrows in the cephalad levels, with one study finding no evident posterior epidural space above C7-T1.[15] For this reason, many practitioners choose to

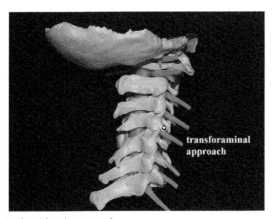

Fig. 2. Transforaminal epidural approach.

perform interlaminar injections at the T1-T2, C7-T1, or C6-C7 interspace with or without the use of a catheter.

Transforaminal Cervical Epidural Injections

The transforaminal approach has a theoretical advantage over the interlaminar technique, as it allows for placement of medication in the anterior epidural space near the targeted spinal nerve and dorsal root ganglion. This advantage needs to be weighed against the increased risk of the procedure, as there have been reports of catastrophic outcomes after cervical transforaminal injections, such as infarction resulting in neurologic deficits, anterior spinal artery syndrome, quadriparesis, brainstem herniation, and even death. There have been 2 studies showing no major complications after cervical interlaminar epidural injections.[16,17] One prospective study with 89 patients showed that 91% of patients had no complications or side effects following cervical transforaminal injections, and a case series of 1036 injections showed no catastrophic complications.[18,19]

One theoretical mechanism behind these adverse events is the possible injection of particulate steroids into the cervical arterial vasculature, resulting in infarction. If a transforaminal approach is to be used, the risks can be minimized by considering the use of a local anesthetic test dose, digital subtraction, real-time live fluoroscopy while injecting contrast, and using a steroid solution with minimal particulate size. There have been no serious events reported after the use of nonparticulate steroids and research has shown that nonparticulate steroids and particulate steroids can both show significant improvements in pain scores 4 weeks after an injection.[20]

Cervical Selective Nerve Root Injections

Selective nerve root blocks are used to target a specific spinal nerve, nerve root, and dorsal root ganglion using a small amount of local anesthetic and to determine the amount of pain relief after the procedure. The technique and utility of selective injections have been controversial. Some practitioners advocate the use of a double-blind, triple-block protocol with injections done with saline, short-acting local anesthetic, and a long-acting local anesthetic in an attempt to improve the accuracy of these blocks. The selective nerve root block uses the transforaminal approach, but injecting only a small amount of local anesthetic to limit the area of nerve block. Therefore, selective nerve root injections theoretically carry the same risks as transforaminal injections. The decision to pursue selective nerve root injections depends on the practitioner, patient comfort, and, if used for surgical planning, surgeon preference.

CERVICAL ZYGAPOPHYSEAL (FACET) JOINT INJECTIONS

Percutaneous interventional treatments have become a valuable and effective tool in helping to diagnose and treat cervical facet joint mediated pain. Cervical facet or zygapophyseal joint disease is a challenging and pervasive entity to treat. A study of 500 patients with chronic cervical spinal pain revealed a prevalence of 55% of patients with facet mediated pain. This finding was determined by injecting 1% lidocaine or 0.25% bupivacaine local anesthetic to the medial branches of the affected zygapophyseal joints. A positive response was defined as at least an 80% reduction of pain with facet loading maneuvers performed after the procedure.[21] This study supports the notion that the posterior elements of the cervical spine can contribute significantly to axial cervical pain.

The zygapophyseal joint is a diarthrodial synovial joint with a fibrous capsule that is heavily innervated by mechanoreceptors. When stimulated with a needle, mass effect from injectate, or mechanical aggravation with facet loading maneuvers, the zygapophyseal joint is capable of manifesting as pure axial spinal pain or transmitting as referred or radicular-like pain. Several studies have established the prevalence of pain patterns from particular joints. One such study revealed pain patterns of joints at segments C2-3 through C6-7. Using fluoroscopic guidance, individual facets joints were injected and aggravated by distending the joint capsules with contrast medium. Each joint stimulated produced a clinically distinct pain pattern essentially creating a cervical facet pain map.[22] These patterns are discussed in further detail by one of the study author in an article by Nikolai Bogduk elsewhere in this issue. These established patterns, along with a thorough history, physical examination, and imaging studies can eliminate an arbitrary approach to treating cervical facet disease with interventional therapy.

Injections to these pain-sensitive structures have revealed both clinically diagnostic and potentially therapeutic value. If more than one pain generator is suspected, successful response to facet injections can help to delineate pain that may stem from the intervertebral disc, radiculopathy, stenosis, myofascial pain, or spondylosis. Interventional treatments for facet-mediated pain in the cervical spine include but are not limited to intraarticular synovial facet injections, diagnostic medial branch blocks, and therapeutic radiofrequency ablation to the medial branches of the cervical dorsal rami that innervate the zygapophyseal joint (**Figs. 3** and **4**).

Intraarticular Zygapophyseal (Facet) Joint Injections

Fluoroscopically guided intraarticular zygapophyseal joint injections are employed after conservative measures have failed and pain is still persistent after passage of time expected for tissue healing. When indicated, these interventions can provide both diagnostic information and therapeutic relief.

A typical zygapophyseal joint with an intact capsule can generally hold anywhere between 1.0 to 1.5 mL of injectate. The capacity of the zygapophyseal joint should be considered to prevent damage or rupture of the capsule and unwanted spread of the injectate into surrounding structures or the epidural space. Because injectate is typically a mixture of a corticosteroid and anesthetic, anesthetic leakage to other neuroaxial pain generators may result in a false-positive response. The injection is usually performed with patients in a prone or lateral decubitus position. The joint line is visualized by fluoroscopy and a gun-barrel approach is taken to direct the spinal needle into the joint. Once the needle tip has penetrated the joint capsule and reached os, a small amount of contrast should be injected to confirm needle placement.

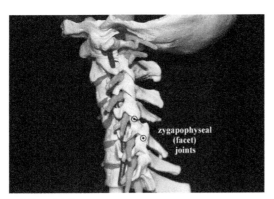

Fig. 3. Zygapophyseal (facet) joints.

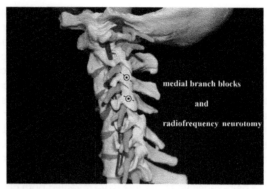

Fig. 4. Medial branch nerves.

Injection of contrast or injectate may induce a pain response and the physician should carefully note whether the pain is concordant with the patients' typical symptoms, as that information may help aid in diagnostic interpretation. Possible complications of facet injections include but are not limited to rupture of the joint capsule and puncture of the vertebral artery or vein, the ventral ramus of the spinal nerve, the epidural space, or even the spinal cord.

Individuals can develop symptomatic synovial cysts (outpocketing of the facet joint synovium) with progressive degeneration of the cervical facet joints. Synovial cysts can invade into the central canal or foraminal space and cause radicular symptoms. These cysts are typically located adjacent to the joint and can be seen as rounded areas of increased signal intensity on T2-weighted magnetic resonance imaging.

Cervical Medial Branch Blocks

The rationale behind the cervical medial branch block is to provide support for a diagnosis of the zygapophyseal joint as the pain generator. Medial branch nerves supply the afferent sensory pain response from the cervical zygapophyseal joint. Successful anesthetic block should interrupt the afferent pain signal of facet-mediated pain and result in relief of pain. The medial branch block is performed as a precursor to radiofrequency medial branch neurotomy, in which a controlled nonsurgical heat lesion made with a radiofrequency probe. Technically, because cervical medial branch blocks have a larger target area and are further away from the neural structures of the cervical spine than intraartciular facet joint injections, it is thought to be easier to perform and felt by some to be theoretically safer. There is less likelihood of entering the epidural space, intervertebral foramen, and vertebral artery when performing medial branch blocks as opposed to intraarticular facet joint injections. However, intraarticular joint injections may be used therapeutically, whereas medial branch nerve blocks are typically used as a purely diagnostic tool.

The nerve supplies to the facet joints are the medial branches derived from the dorsal primary rami of the nerve root. The C2-3 joint is innervated by 2 branches of the dorsal rami: the communicating branch and a medial branch known as the third occipital nerve. The C3-4 through C7-T1 joints are supplied by the dorsal rami medial branches. The anatomy is such that 2 medial branches supply 1 joint. For example, the C5-6 zygapophyseal joint is innervated by both the C5 and C6 medial branches at the respective C5 and C6 articular pillars (further discussion regarding facet joint anatomy, innervation, and pain is covered in an article by Nikolai Bogduk elsewhere in this issue). Therefore, it is inadequate to block only 1 medial branch for any given joint as it only blocks half the joint and precludes symptom relief.

Typically any preservative-free local anesthetic can be used. The most commonly used agents include bupivacaine and lidocaine with varying concentrations. Because small volumes are recommended, no more than 0.3 mL per nerve for adequate blockade, high concentrations offer the most anesthetic response.[23]

Successful blockade of the medial branch block per practice guidelines have suggested that complete relief of pain in a distinct pattern that correlate to the nerves being anaesthetized should be achieved to proceed to percutaneous radiofrequency neurotomy.[23]

Radiofrequency Neurotomy (Ablation)

Radiofrequency neurotomy of the medial branches is a useful modality to help treat confirmed facetogenic pain. The procedure was first described in 1974 when it was used by Shealy in the treatment of lumbar spinal pain.[24] The procedure is performed with a Teflon-coated electrode in which the tip remains exposed to generate a high-frequency electrical current to thermocoagulate the medial branch nerves. This procedure disrupts nociceptive conduction from the painful facet joint. Proper patient selection is paramount to achieve successful outcome. The appropriate patients for the procedure have had demonstrated improvement in pain with either intraarticular zygapophyseal joint injections or medial branch blocks. Neither prior surgery nor prior radiofrequency ablation precludes patients from undergoing the procedure.

In a randomized, double-blind trial, 24 subjects who had been determined to have zygapophyseal joint-mediated pain underwent radiofrequency neurotomy with a control group that received needle placement without electrical thermocoagulation. The results revealed that the median duration of relief was 263 days (almost 9 months) in the active-treatment group before their pain returned to 50% of the preprocedure level.[25] Pain relief from radiofrequency neurotomy can be long lasting, but as the medial branches grow back the pain may return and a repeat radiofrequency may be needed. Another study determining the long-term efficacy of radiofrequency neurotomy evaluated 28 patients who were involved in a motor vehicle accident and revealed complete relief in 71% of patients after the procedure. The pain relief lasted a mean duration of 422 days after the first procedure and 219 days after the repeat procedure.[26]

Serious complications from radiofrequency neurotomy can be avoided if the procedure is performed correctly. Theoretical risks that exist for most spinal interventions still apply. Adverse neurologic side effects reported with radiofrequency neurotomy of medial branches from C3 through C7 include vasovagal syncope, dermoid cyst, neuritis, numbness in the cutaneous region of the denervated nerve, and dysesthesias in the cutaneous region of the denervated nerve. Postdenervation neuritis and numbness have been the most reported side effect and fortunately are usually short lived with spontaneous resolution of these symptoms occurring without treatment between 1 to 6 weeks after the onset of symptoms.[23]

Another consideration with radiofrequency neurotomy is that a portion of the cervical paraspinal musculature can be denervated. The deeper cervical paraspinal muscles are innervated by the same dorsal rami targeted for neurotomy; some authors have even used electromyography to confirm a successful procedure.[27] Although serious complications are rare, there has been report of spinal cord injury from radiofrequency neurotomy. A patient developed a Brown-Sequard syndrome following a C3-4 radiofrequency neurotomy, in which the radiofrequency needle was placed medial to the laminae and was advanced into the spinal cord causing a thermocoagulation lesion of the cord. The patient could not report adverse response during the procedure because they were under general anesthesia.[2]

Pulsed radiofrequency neurotomy has been used more recently to help minimize the risk of adverse events. This technique involves placing a standard Teflon-coated radiofrequency needle at the precise anatomic location of the medial branch but using significantly lower temperatures to coagulate the nerve. Current studies suggest a significantly lower side-effect profile with pulsed radiofrequency neurotomy versus conventional radiofrequency. A study of 114 patients who had positive response to diagnostic blocks underwent pulsed radiofrequency lesion at 42°C for 120 seconds. The results revealed that 46 patients did not respond favorably to pulsed radiofrequency neurotomy (pain reduction <50%) and 68 patients had a successful response with an average of 3.93 ± 1.86 months. Eighteen of these 68 patients went on to have the procedure repeated. Although small, this study showed that pulsed radiofrequency neurotomy to medial branches of the dorsal rami in patients with chronic zygapophyseal joint arthropathy provided temporary pain relief in 59.6% of patients.[28] Thus, although pulsed radiofrequency neurotomy is theoretically safer, it may not have the same efficacy as that of conventional radiofrequency neurotomy.

NEUROMODULATION: SPINAL CORD STIMULATION

Spinal cord stimulation was first described in 1967 as a treatment method for pain.[29] Since then it has been used to treat various painful conditions, including angina, complex regional pain syndrome, neuropathic pain syndromes, and radiculopathy. Although the mechanism of action is poorly understood, there has been research that shows that spinal cord stimulation may cause changes to the local chemical composition of the dorsal horn, with increased γ-aminobutyric acid and serotonin release, as well as possible suppression of glutamate and aspartate.

The procedure involves placing electrodes near the dorsal column of the spinal cord to modulate pain. The area of paresthesia produced by the electrode must overlap the area of pain and the selection of levels stimulated is based on dermatomal representation of the painful area. As such, patient feedback during the procedure is imperative to ensure coverage of painful area. Technology has evolved to allow for various current, voltage, waveform, and lead/electrode configurations. Traditionally, limitations of spinal cord stimulation for cervical pain have been caused by increased migration of electrodes in the cervical spine. Because the cervical spine has more motion than the thoracic spine, where leads for lumbar pain are typically placed, percutaneous lead migration can be problematic. With the advent of laminotomy paddle leads, this problem has been addressed and more patients are undergoing spinal cord stimulation for cervical pain.[30,31] Paddle leads have been shown to be superior to percutaneous leads in terms of migration rate, and retrograde placement of paddle leads from C1-C2 has been described as being safe and effective for cervical pain and neuropathic pain syndromes of the upper extremity.[32]

One of the most important factors in predicting successful outcome is patient selection. The spinal cord stimulator procedure is performed in 2 steps: trial, and if successful, subsequent implantation. After patients are deemed appropriate candidates for spinal cord stimulation by undergoing a psychological evaluation and proper education, patients undergo a percutaneous lead trial for 3 to 7 days to assess the efficacy of the stimulator in improving their pain. If the trial is successful and patients choose to proceed with the implant, referral to a surgeon can be made for a paddle lead implant. Complications from spinal cord stimulators range from infection, hematomas, and cerebrospinal fluid leaks to paralysis, nerve injury, and death.[33] For patients with failed back surgery syndrome, who may not be surgical candidates or who do not wish to undergo spine surgery, spinal cord stimulation may be an attractive and cost-effective option.[34] A study looking at the effectiveness of spinal cord stimulation of the cervical spine showed that 68% of patients had sustained pain relief with median follow-up of 4 years and 7 months.[35]

DISCUSSION

Cervical interventional procedures, if used appropriately by properly trained physicians and in carefully selected patients, can be useful in aiding the diagnosis of painful structures and for providing symptomatic relief to patients who have failed conservative treatment methods. Physiatrists, with their extensive training in neurologic and musculoskeletal anatomy, history taking and physical examination techniques, the use of electrodiagnostic testing when appropriate, and the interpretation of radiographic findings in the clinical context, are ideally positioned to provide a sophisticated and efficient method of controlling pain and restoring function. Interventional techniques can be employed with patient education and therapy to help maximize symptom relief and potentiate long-term changes. It is important to improve the current state of research about cervical pain and treatment, and to reduce pain-related disability for those with conditions impairing their function and quality of life. Image-guided injections, radiofrequency techniques, neuromodulation, and exploration of other injectates, such as stem cells, all hold promise for nonsurgical treatment of cervical pain.

REFERENCES

1. Horlocker TT, Wedel DJ, Rowlingson JC, et al. Regional anesthesia in the patient receiving antithrombotic or thrombolytic therapy: American Society of Regional Anesthesia and Pain Medicine evidence-based guidelines (third edition). Reg Anesth Pain Med 2010;35:64–101.
2. Bogduk N. Complications of spinal diagnostic and treatment procedures. Pain Med 2008;9:S12–31.
3. Ferrante FM, Wilson SP, Iacobo C, et al. Clinical classification as a predictor of therapeutic outcome after cervical epidural steroid injection. Spine 1993;18: 730–6.
4. Johansson A, Hao J, Sjolund B. Local corticosteroid application blocks transmission in normal nociceptive C-fibers. Acta Anaesthesiol Scand 1990;34:335–8.
5. Hua SY, Chen YZ. Membrane receptor-mediated electrophysiological effects of glucocorticoid on mammalian neurons. Endocrinology 1989;124:687–91.
6. Bush K, Hillier S. Outcome of cervical radiculopathy treated with periradicular epidural corticosteroid injections: a prospective study with independent clinical review. Eur Spine J 1996;5:319–25.
7. Slipman CW, Lipetz JS, Jackson HB, et al. Therapeutic selective nerve root block in the nonsurgical treatment of atraumatic cervical spondylotic radicular pain: a retrospective analysis with independent clinical review. Arch Phys Med Rehabil 2000;81:741–6.
8. Cyteval C, Thomas E, Pecoux E, et al. Cervical radiculopathy: open study on percutaneous periradicular foraminal steroid infiltration performed under CT control in 30 patients. AJNR Am J Neuroradiol 2004;25:441–5.
9. Benyamin RM, Singh V, Parr AT, et al. Systematic review of the effectiveness of cervical epidurals in the management of chronic neck pain. Pain Physician 2009;12(1):137–57.

10. Bloomberg RG, Joanivald A, Walther S. Advantages of the paramedian approach for lumbar epidural analgesia with catheter technique. A clinical comparison between midline and paramedian approaches. Anaesthesia 1989;44:742–6.

11. Stojanovic MP, Vu T, Caneris O, et al. The role of fluoroscopy in cervical epidural steroid injections. An analysis of contrast dispersal patterns. Spine 2002;27: 509–14.

12. Renfew DL, Moore TE, Kathol MH. Correct placement of epidural steroid injections: fluoroscopic guidance and contrast administration. AJNR Am J Neuroradiol 1991;12:1003–7.

13. Sullivan WJ, Willick SE, Chira-Adisai W, et al. Incidence of intravascular uptake in lumbar spinal injection procedures. Spine 2000;25:481–6.

14. Furman MB, O'Brien EM, Zgleszewski TM. Incidence of intravascular penetration in transforaminal lumbosacral epidural steroid injections. Spine 2000;25:2628–32.

15. Hogan QH. Epidural anatomy examined by cryomicrotome section. Reg Anesth 1996;21:395–406.

16. Johnson BA, Schellhas KP, Pollei SR. Epidurography and therapeutic epidural injections: technical considerations and experience with 5334 cases. AJNR Am J Neuroradiol 1999;20:697–705.

17. Botwin KP, Castellanos R, Raos, et al. Complications of fluoroscopically guided interlaminar cervical injections. Arch Phys Med Rehabil 2003;84:627–33.

18. Huston CW, Slipman CW, Garvin C. Complications and side effect of cervical and lumbosacral selective nerve root injections. Arch Phys Med Rehabil 2005;86: 277–83.

19. Ma DJ, Gilula LA, Riew KD. Complications of fluoroscopically guided extraforaminal cervical nerve root blocks. An analysis of 1036 injections. J Bone Joint Surg Am 2005;87:1025–30.

20. Dreyfuss P, Baker R, Bogduk N. Comparative effectiveness of cervical transforaminal injections with particulate and nonparticulate corticosteroid preparations for cervical radicular pain. Pain Med 2006;7:237–42.

21. Manchikati L. Prevalence of facet joint in chronic spinal pain of cervical, thoracic, and lumbar regions. BMC Musculoskelet Disord 2004;5:15.

22. Dwyer A, Aprill C, Bogduk N. Cervical zygapophyseal joint pain patterns I: a study in normal volunteers. Spine 1990;15:458–61.

23. Bogduk N, editor. Practice guidelines for spinal diagnostic and treatment procedures. San Francisco (CA): Library of Congress Cataloging in Publication Data; 2004.

24. Shealy CN. Percutaneous radiofrequency denervation of spinal facets. J Neurosurg 1975;43:448–51.

25. Lord SM, Barnsley L, Wallis BJ, et al. Percutaneous radiofrequency neurotomy for chronic cervical zygapophyseal-joint pain. N Engl J Med 1996;335(23): 1721–6.

26. McDonald GJ, Lord SM, Bogduk N. Long term follow-up of patients treated with cervical radiofrequency neurotomy for chronic neck pain. Neurosurgery 1999; 45(1):61–7.

27. Oudenhoven RC. Paraspinal electromyography following facet rhizotomy. Spine 1977;2:299–304.

28. Mikeladze G, Espinal R, Finnegan R, et al. Pulsed radiofrequency application in treatment of chronic zygapophyseal joint pain. Spine J 2003;3(5):360–2.

29. Shealy CN, Mortimer JT, Reswick JB. Electrical inhibition of pain by stimulation of the dorsal columns: preliminary clinical report. Anesth Analg 1967;46:489–91.

30. Barolat G. Experience with 509 plate-electrodes implanted epidurally from C1 to L1. Stereotact Funct Neurosurg 1993;61:60–79.
31. Villavicencio AT, Leveque JC, Rubin L, et al. Laminectomy versus percutaneous electrode placement for spinal cord stimulation. Neurosurgery 2000;46:399–405.
32. Whitworth LA, Feler CA. C1–C2 Sublaminar insertion of paddle leads for the management of chronic painful conditions of the upper extremity. Neuromodulation 2003;6(3):153–7.
33. Linderoth B, Foreman R. "Physiology of spinal cord stimulation: review and update". Neuromodulation 1999;3:150–64.
34. Kumar K, Malik S, Demeria D. "Treatment of chronic pain with spinal cord stimulation versus alternative therapies: cost-effectiveness analysis". Neurosurgery 2002;51(1):106–15.
35. Simpson BA, Gill B, Davies K, et al. Cervical spinal cord stimulation for pain: a report on 41 patients. Neuromodulation 2003;6(1):20–6.

Neck Pain from a Spine Surgeon's Perspective

Rahul Basho, MD[a],*, Amandeep Bhalla, MD[b], Jeffrey C. Wang, MD[c]

KEYWORDS

• Neck pain • Radiculopathy • Spondylosis • Myelopathy
• Spine surgery

Through the myriad of abnormalities encountered by spine surgeons, neck pain is one of the most perplexing. The nature, onset, and location of the pain all provide information as to what the potential pain generator may be. By synthesizing data garnered from the physical examination, imaging studies, and history, a spine surgeon must formulate a differential diagnosis and treatment plan. The surgeon must determine whether the patient has cervical radiculopathy, myelopathy, or simply cervical spondylosis because the treatment of each of these is vastly different.

CERVICAL SPONDYLOSIS

Generalized arthropathy of the cervical spine, or cervical spondylosis, results in hypertrophied facets, bone spurs, and degeneration of the disks. Although the contribution of each of these to the patient's symptoms has not been elucidated, nociceptive pain endings have been found in the peripheral portions of the disk and in the capsule and synovium of the facet joints.[1–4] Patients typically present with neck pain that is not radicular in nature. Physicians must be cognizant of the upper cervical dermatomes, such as the upper shoulder and trapezial areas, realizing that pain in these distributions may represent referred or radicular pain. In addition, other causes of neck pain, such as cervical instability, must be ruled out with flexion-extension radiographs.

Once the physical examination and imaging studies determine that the patient has cervical spondylosis, extensive conservative management should be initiated. Use of nonsteroidal antiinflammatory drugs (NSAIDs), muscle relaxants, and other analgesics is the common first-line treatment option. In addition, a 4- to 6-week course of

The authors have nothing to disclose.
[a] Riverside County Regional Medical Center, Riverside, CA 92507, USA
[b] Department of Orthopaedic Surgery, Harbor - University of California Los Angeles Medical Center, 1000 West Carson Street, Torrance, CA, USA
[c] UCLA Spine Center, UCLA School of Medicine, 1250 16th Street, Suite 745, Santa Monica, CA 90404, USA
* Corresponding author.
E-mail address: rbasho@haiderspine.com

physical therapy should be initiated. Studies have shown that a physical therapy regimen that includes isometric and active strengthening, active range of motion, and aerobic conditioning has beneficial effects in patients with chronic neck pain.[5,6] Other conservative modalities, such as heat and cold therapy, transcutaneous electrical nerve stimulation units, and cervical traction, were not shown to have any reproducible benefit in a recent meta-analysis of the literature.[7]

Persistent pain in patients despite a 6-month course of conservative management is a difficult diagnostic dilemma for surgeons. Because of the paucity of prospective randomized controlled studies examining the success rates of cervical fusions for axial neck pain, most surgeons are hesitant to offer this as a treatment option. Surgical success rates seem to improve when preoperative diskography is used to localize symptomatic levels. Palit and colleagues[8] performed anterior cervical fusions on patients with axial neck pain who had positive results of diskograms. This prospective study on 38 patients showed that approximately 80% of the patients were satisfied with the surgical outcome and underscored the importance of preoperative provocative diskography when performing cervical fusions for axial neck pain. Whitecloud and Seago[9] also performed anterior cervical fusions for axial neck pain and reported good outcomes in 70% of the patients. However, this study was retrospective, had 85% follow-up, and did not use quantitative outcome criteria.[9,10] Despite the lack of definitive data, the overall trends have resulted in most physicians obtaining preoperative diskograms in patients with axial neck pain to better delineate the pain generator and minimize the number of levels fused.

Provocative discography is performed by injecting a water-soluble radiopaque dye under fluoroscopic guidance into an intervertebral disk. It is used to confirm the diagnosis of internal disk disruption and demonstrate the presence of normal disks adjacent to the level of an intended spinal fusion. Its role as an evaluative procedure is based on whether the disk injection reproduces the patient's neck pain. The distribution and presence of dye extravasation are also noted. The patient's pain intensity is measured on a standardized scale, and the concordance of the pain caused by the diskogram with the patient's original presenting pain is also rated. A control disk injection is often performed to add validity to the study and must have a negative result to declare the diskogram positive.

There are many challenges with the evaluative quality of provocative discography. Differentiating pain caused by the injection from the patient's baseline neck pain can be difficult and confounded by patients with regional pain that does not originate from the intervertebral disk. Furthermore, the patient's own neurophysiologic modulation of pain pathways, which may amplify or downregulate nociceptive signals from the injected disk, affects the subjective reporting of pain perception on which the procedure relies. Factors commonly reported to increase the risk of false-positive results of injections include patients with increased psychological distress, concurrent chronic pain syndromes, disputed compensation claims, previous diskectomy at the injected disk, and a history of persistent clinically benign backache.[11]

In addition to the controversy surrounding the evaluative efficacy of diskography in patients with degenerative disk disease and severe neck pain, there are risks associated with the procedure. The literature has reported risk for diskitis, subdural empyema, spinal cord injury, vascular injury, and prevertebral abscess formation. In a retrospective analysis of 4400 cervical disk injections in 1357 patients, Zeidman and colleagues[12] reported significant complications from the procedure in less than 0.6% of the patients and 0.16% of cervical disk injections. Of the 4400 injections, 7 were complicated by diskitis, with patients presenting within a week after diskography complaining of acute exacerbation of mechanical cervical pain without a radicular component. Two of these patients reported low-grade febrile episodes. Other complications included prevertebral abscess and symptomatic disk space infections.

Patients with axial neck pain who fail conservative therapy should be considered for provocative diskography. If the result of the diskogram is positive, surgery in the form of a fusion can be offered to the patient. The patient must be counseled that even with a positive result of diskography, surgery for axial neck pain is not backed by strong scientific data.

CERVICAL RADICULOPATHY

According to the most recent North American Spine Society (NASS) guidelines, cervical radiculopathy is defined as "pain in a radicular pattern in one or both upper extremities related to compression and/or irritation of one or more cervical nerve roots." Patients will present with "varying degrees of sensory, motor, and reflex changes without evidence of spinal cord dysfunction (myelopathy)." As the cervical disks gradually lose height, they can bulge posteriorly and impinge on the nerve within the neuroforamina. Loss of disk height also narrows the foramen, causes the ligamentum flavum to become redundant, and places increased stresses on the facet joints. The increased stress results in osteophyte formation in both the facets and uncovertebral joints, causing further narrowing in the neuroforamen.

The natural history of cervical radiculopathy has been extensively studied and traditionally been described as favorable. Cervical radiculopathy caused by disk herniations spontaneously resolves in approximately 95% of cases.[13] The NASS guidelines for the management of cervical radiculopathy, however, are less conclusive. Citing limitations of available literature, the work group was unable to definitively comment on the natural history of cervical radiculopathy from degenerative disorders. The guidelines state, unspecifically, that "it is likely that for most patients with cervical radiculopathy from degenerative disorders signs and symptoms will be self-limited and will resolve spontaneously over a variable length of time without specific treatment."

Initial treatment of cervical radiculopathy should be conservative. The same modalities used to treat cervical spondylosis, such as NSAIDs, analgesics, and physical therapy, should be initiated. Epidural steroid injections may be used for both diagnostic and therapeutic purposes.

Failure of conservative management, a worsening neurologic deficit, and intractable pain are all indications for surgical intervention. The anatomic location of the patient's herniation helps determine the type of surgical intervention. Patients with unilateral radicular symptoms, no evidence of instability on flexion-extension radiographs, and unilateral radicular symptoms with a far-lateral herniation on magnetic resonance imaging (MRI) can be treated with a posterior cervical foraminotomy. This procedure avoids fusing a segment of the cervical spine and can be done through a small incision. However, it is not indicated for patients with compression from uncovertebral joint hypertrophy, the so-called hard disk herniations.[14]

Patients with central or paracentral herniations on MRI with either unilateral or bilateral radicular findings can be treated with an anterior cervical diskectomy and fusion. Through an anterior approach, both neuroforamina can be decompressed. The disk is removed entirely and replaced with a cage with either autograft or allograft. Up to 3 cervical levels can be decompressed in this manner with good fusion rates, but decompressing more levels will require supplemental posterior fixation. Clinical results for anterior cervical diskectomy and fusion have shown good to excellent results in 70% to 90% of patients.[15–17] Factors not associated with the clinical outcome include the age of the patient and type of disk herniation (soft or hard). Male gender, greater segmental kyphosis, and a low score on the Neck Disability Index have been associated with better clinical outcomes.[18]

CERVICAL MYELOPATHY

Mechanical compression of the spinal cord results in cervical myelopathy. Patients typically present with gait abnormalities and difficulty with fine motor movements of the hands and also often have some degree of axial neck pain and radiculopathy. Common physical examination findings include hyperreflexia, clonus, and the presence of abnormal reflexes (Hoffman or Babinski reflex). Patients will often have difficulty with tandem gait and state that they have been falling or feel unsteady on their feet.

As with other conditions involving neck pain, initial radiographs should include anteroposterior, lateral, and flexion-extension radiographs of the cervical spine. The presence of gross instability on dynamic views can indicate pressure on the spinal cord with motion. MRI is the diagnostic standard for evaluating the status of the disks, nerves, and intramedullary substance of the spinal cord. A hyperintense signal in the substance of the spinal cord isolated on T2-weighted images indicates inflammation and edema, which may resolve. A combination of low signal intensity on T1-weighted images and high signal intensity on T2-weighted images indicates more severe damage to the spinal cord and is typically found in the later stages of cervical myelopathy.[19]

Classic studies on the natural history of cervical myelopathy have shown that its course is one of a stepwise decline.[20] Patients will have periods of stable function followed by instances of precipitous decline. For this reason, surgeons are typically more aggressive when treating patients with myelopathy. If conservative treatment is initiated, close follow-up of patients is needed. Patients must have a clear understanding that further neurologic decline may not be recoverable.

Surgical intervention for cervical myelopathy involves decompression of the spinal cord, through either an anterior or a posterior approach. Both necessitate a fusion and have yielded excellent results. Newer techniques such as laminoplasty have been used more widely. Laminoplasty preserves cervical motion by hinging open the laminae, thereby increasing the space available for the cord without a fusion. If patients have minimal neck pain, laminoplasty is also an option and has yielded similar outcomes.[21]

Spine surgeons must have a systematic approach to patients with neck pain and obtain a thorough history and physical examination. By correlating this information with plain radiographs and magnetic resonance images, surgeons can formulate a treatment plan and counsel the patient as to the likely outcomes. Newer techniques such as laminoplasty show promising results and give surgeons another arrow in their quiver. Other questions, such as the efficacy of surgery for axial neck pain, need better data with randomized prospective studies. As the knowledge of the anatomy, pain generators, and intricate dynamics of the spine continues to progress, so will the surgeons' ability to bring relief and succor to his or her patients.

REFERENCES

1. Ferlic DC. The nerve supply of the cervical intervertebral disc in man. Bull Johns Hopkins Hosp 1963;113:347–51.
2. McLain RF. Mechanoreceptor endings in human cervical facet joints. Spine 1994; 19:495–501.

3. Chen C, Lu Y, Kallakuri S, et al. Distribution of A-delta and C-fiber receptors in the cervical facet joint capsule and their response to stretch. J Bone Joint Surg Am 2006;88:1807–16.
4. Inami S, Shiga T, Tsujino A, et al. Immunohistochemical demonstration of nerve fibers in the synovial fold of the human cervical facet joint. J Orthop Res 2001; 19:593–6.
5. Wang WT, Olson SL, Campbell AH, et al. Effectiveness of physical therapy for patients with neck pain: an individualized approach using a clinical decision-making algorithm. Am J Phys Med Rehabil 2003;82:203–21.
6. Chiu TT, Lam TH, Hedley AJ. A randomized controlled trial on the efficacy of exercise for patients with chronic neck pain. Spine 2005;30:E1–7.
7. Philadelphia Panel. Philadelphia panel evidence-based clinical practice guidelines on selected rehabilitation interventions for neck pain. Phys Ther 2001;81: 1701–17.
8. Palit M, Schofferman J, Goldthwaite N, et al. Anterior discectomy and fusion for the management of neck pain. Spine 1999;24:2224–8.
9. Whitecloud TS, Seago RA. Cervical discogenic syndrome: results of operative intervention in patients with positive discography. Spine 1987;12:313–6.
10. Siebenrock KA, Aebi M. [The value of discography in disc-related pain syndrome of the cervical spine for evaluation of indications for spondylodesis]. Z Orthop Ihre Grenzgeb 1993;131:220–4 [in German].
11. Tornetta P, Einhorn T. Orthopaedic surgery essentials: Spine. Philadelphia: Lippincott Williams & Wilkins; 2004.
12. Zeidman S, Thompson K, Ducker T. Complications of cervical discography: analysis of 4400 diagnostic disc injections. Neurosurgery 1995;37:414–7.
13. Spivak J, Connolly P. Orthopedic knowledge update: Spine 3. Rosemont (IL): American Academy of Orthopedic Surgeons; 2006. p. 228–34.
14. Russell SM, Benjamin V. Posterior surgical approach to the cervical neural foramen for intervertebral disc disease. Neurosurgery 2004;54:662–6.
15. Bohlman HH, Emery SE, Goodfellow DB, et al. Robinson anterior cervical discectomy and arthrodesis for cervical radiculopathy. Long-term follow-up of one hundred and twenty-two patients. J Bone Joint Surg Am 1993;75:1298–307.
16. Gore DR, Sepic SB. Anterior cervical fusion for degenerated or protruded discs. A review of one hundred forty-six patients. Spine 1984;9:667–71.
17. Goldberg EJ, Singh K, Van U, et al. Comparing outcomes of anterior cervical discectomy and fusion in workman's versus non-workman's compensation population. Spine J 2002;2:408–14.
18. Peolsson A, Hedlund R, Vavruch L, et al. Predictive factors for the outcome of anterior cervical decompression and fusion. Eur Spine J 2003;12:274–80.
19. Wada E, Ohmura M, Yonenobu K. Intramedullary changes of the spinal cord in cervical spondylotic myelopathy. Spine 1995;20:2226–32.
20. Nurick S. The natural history and the results of surgical treatment of the spinal cord disorder associated with cervical spondylosis. Brain 1972;95:101–8.
21. Wada E, Suzuki S, Kanazawa A, et al. Subtotal corpectomy versus laminoplasty for multilevel cervical spondylotic myelopathy: a long-term follow-up study over 10 years. Spine 2001;26:1443–8.

Index

Note: Page numbers of article titles are in **boldface** type.

A

Acetaminophen, in neck pain, 505–506
Acupuncture, chi and, 524
 for mechanical neck disorders, 525
 in neck pain, 524–525
 safety of, 525
Adson test, 477, 478
Analgesics, topical, in neck pain, 509–510
Ankylosing hyperostosis. See *Skeletal hyperostosis, diffuse idiopathic.*
Ankylosing spondylitis, back pain in, 487
 chest wall expansion in, 488
 delay in diagnosis of, 488
 extra-articular complications of, 489
 laboratory assessment of, 488
 spinal fractures and, 423
 treatment of, 489
Antiepileptic drugs, in neck pain, 508
Arthropathies, inflammatory, neck pain in, 375
Athlete, competitive, cervical spine pain in, **459–471**
Atlantoaxial disease, in rheumatoid arthritis, 420, 421
Atlantoaxial instability, conditions associated with, 419–422, 423
 in Down syndrome, 468–469
Atlantoaxial subluxation, in rheumatoid arthritis, 420, 421, 486

B

Botulinum toxin, in neck pain, 510
Burners, in athletes, 462–463

C

Canadian C-Spine Rules, trauma patients and, 413, 414
Capsaicin, topical, in neck pain, 509
Capsular strain, facet joint whiplash injury and, 453–454
Cervical canal stenosis, 390
Cervical cord neuropraxia, in athlete, 463–464
Cervical facet arthrosis, 390
Cervical facet-mediated pain, **447–458**
 diagnostic injections in, 451
 differential diagnosis of, 451
Cervical pain, cervical epidural injections in, 540–542
 cervical zygapophyseal (facet) joint injections in, 542–546
 interventional procedures for, **539–549**

Phys Med Rehabil Clin N Am 22 (2011) 557–564
doi:10.1016/S1047-9651(11)00067-2
1047-9651/11/$ – see front matter © 2011 Elsevier Inc. All rights reserved.

pmr.theclinics.com

Moving?

Make sure your subscription moves with you!

To notify us of your new address, find your **Clinics Account Number** (located on your mailing label above your name), and contact customer service at:

Email: journalscustomerservice-usa@elsevier.com

800-654-2452 (subscribers in the U.S. & Canada)
314-447-8871 (subscribers outside of the U.S. & Canada)

Fax number: 314-447-8029

Elsevier Health Sciences Division
Subscription Customer Service
3251 Riverport Lane
Maryland Heights, MO 63043

*To ensure uninterrupted delivery of your subscription, please notify us at least 4 weeks in advance of move.

Printed and bound by CPI Group (UK) Ltd, Croydon, CR0 4YY

03/10/2024

01040452-0001